The Purification Principle

The Purification Principle

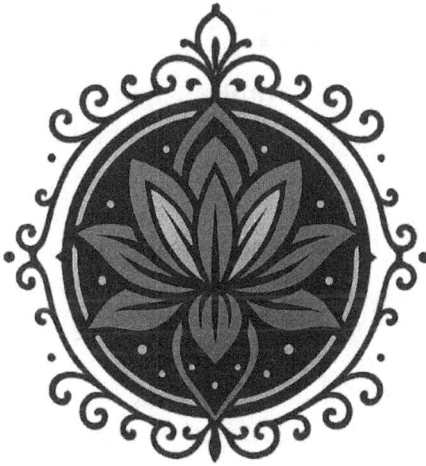

A River Map for Returning to Your Natural State of Health

Co-Authored By:
Jesse J. Jacoby & Sydney Thackray

Soulspire Publishing
Truckee, CA, 96161

ISBN: 978-1-968660-23-9
Library of Congress Control Number: 2012921011
Dewey CIP: 641.563   **OCLC:** 213839254

Cover art, font, and layout are all original art by:

Wholesalers to book trade: Nelson's Books and Ingram
Available through Amazon.com, BarnesAndNoble.com

Dedication

To the rivers that raised us. The clear ones, the clouded ones, and the ones we had to learn to cleanse ourselves.

To every soul who has felt the heaviness of a body out of balance, and to every heart that has longed for a way back to natural clarity.

To the elders, the healers, the teachers, and to the plants, waters, and winds who spoke to us when no one else knew the words.

To our families, who walked beside us in both the still pools and the rapids.

To you, dear reader, for choosing to step into the current, for trusting that your own river can run clear again, and for carrying that clarity into a world that is in need now more than ever.

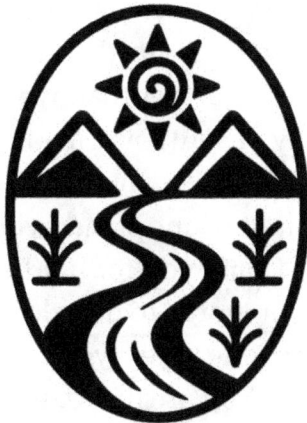

Acknowledgments

This book was not written in isolation. This is the confluence of many rivers, each bringing their own minerals, music, and medicine.

To our families. For the patience, love, and steady presence that made space for this work to flow into being. Your belief in us has been the quiet current carrying us forward.

To the elders and teachers, both living and ancestral, who shared their stories, their plant knowledge, their ceremonies, and their trust. Your wisdom is the bedrock on which these pages rest.

To the healers, guides, and fellow seekers who have walked beside us in purification. In the sweat lodge, in the forest, in the clinic, and in moments of deep personal transformation. You have reminded us that purification is not a solo act, but a collective rising.

To the land. For her beauty, her lessons, and her endless generosity. To the rivers whose waters have cleansed us, the mountains whose silence has steadied us, and the winds that have carried our prayers farther than we could see.

To the community at SoulSpire. Your courage to step into advanced purification, to meet your own depths, and to share your stories has inspired us more than you know.

To every reader. Thank you for holding this book in your hands, for allowing our words to mingle with your own inner waters, and for carrying the work of The Purification Principle into your life. You are the reason we wrote, rewrote, and kept going until the river ran clear.

A Word Before We Begin

Like a river guide pointing to shifting currents, this book offers pathways, not prescriptions. What you will find in these pages is a weaving of personal experience, indigenous wisdom, modern science, and the voice of the land speaking.

This is not intended to diagnose, treat, cure, or prevent disease. We are not your physicians, and this book is not a substitute for personalized medical care. Your body is your own. The currents, depths, and your history. They all belong to you. Before beginning any new practice, cleansing method, dietary change, or advanced therapy, consult with a qualified healthcare provider who can help you navigate safely.

While many of the plants, practices, and modalities described here have been used for generations, each person's river flows differently. What is medicine for one may be a stone for another. Listen inward. Go slowly. Respect your own pace.

If you are pregnant, nursing, taking medications, living with chronic illness, or recovering from injury, you are responsible for seeking professional guidance before diving into any of the deeper waters described.

This book offers knowledge and inspiration. You alone carry the paddle for your own canoe.

Read these words as a companion for your journey, not a replacement for the wise counsel of those who know your health story intimately. Take what resonates, release what does not, and let your own clear waters guide you home.

The River Map Legend

How to read your journey through The Purification Principle

Every river has bends, still pools, and rapids. This map will guide you through the three great movements of The Purification Principle. You can follow them in order or wade in where you feel called. The current will carry you either way.

Movement One: Removing Interference

Symbol: *(Stone in the River)*

Represents the clearing of what does not belong — toxins, stagnant thoughts, heavy emotions, and unseen energetic debris. These are the stones lifted from your riverbed so the water can run free.

Movement Two: Restoring Flow

Symbol: *(Flowing Current)*

Represents reawakening the body's natural rhythms — breath, hydration, movement, seasonal alignment. This is the water moving again, carrying nourishment where it is needed.

Movement Three — Rebuilding Resilience

Symbol: *(Rooted Tree by the Water)*

Represents strengthening foundations. Mitochondria, the microbiome, our nervous system, and emotional stability. This is the riverbank fortified so the flow can endure all seasons.

The River Map

Your guide through the waters of The Purification Principle

Introduction: Where the River Clears

There is a place in the river where the water runs so clearly you can see every stone resting at the bottom. This is the nature of the body when returned to our original state. Nothing clouded. Nothing clinging. The current alive with light.

Purification is not punishment. This is not austerity or the denial of joy. We reference the return of the river to our true, innate nature.

We live in a time where the waters of the earth and body run murky with silt and sorrow. In the villages of our elders, the seasons themselves guided the cleansing. The spring thaw released the winter's weight. Summer's abundance brought fruits that flushed the blood. Autumn taught letting go, and winter offered stillness to integrate the year's medicine. There was no separation between the cycles of the land and cycles of the human being.

The Purification Principle is the remembering of this unity. A way of living that understands the body as a vessel for spirit, the mind as a riverbed for thought, and the heart as the fire that keeps the whole warm. When we remove what does not belong and restore what is essential, the vessel shines, the river runs free, and the fire burns clear.

In the teachings of Alice Bailey, there is the recognition that humanity moves through waves of initiation. Each one requires the leaving behind of old sediment before the next current can be met. Thich Nhat Hanh reminds us that a single mindful breath can wash centuries of dust from the mind. Richard Rudd speaks of the higher frequencies waiting within us, dormant until we clear the lower debris.

Chogyam Trungpa warns that spiritual purity is not a costume but a nakedness, a stripping away until nothing false remains. Deepak Chopra reminds us that every cell listens to the stories we tell, and the story of purity is the story of remembering what we are made of.

The Purification Principle is not a seven-day juice cleanse or a weekend retreat, though these can be included. We are not discussing a temporary escape from the pollution of the modern world, though the principle does offer refuge from this. We are presenting the cultivation of a way of being in which removing interference becomes as natural as exhaling, restoring flow becomes as natural as drinking from a mountain spring, and rebuilding resilience becomes as natural as the forest thickening after a fire.

Our ancestors, both of blood and of spirit, knew this. They sat in the smoke of cedar and sage not because this was tradition, but because the smoke spirits cleared the unseen clutter from the air and the soul. They rose before the sun to greet the day with song, not because they needed ritual for ritual's sake, but because sound and intention reshape the waters within. They fasted when the earth slept, not to impress the gods, but to give the body time to sweep all inner rooms clean.

We are being called to remember these ways. Not as artifacts of a romanticized past, but as living technologies. In this remembering, The Purification Principle becomes more than a philosophy; the teachings become a compass that points to what is essential, discards what is false, and walks us back to the place in the river where the water runs clear.

You will find no dogma here. You will not be told to adopt a single diet, to take on a single spiritual path, or to reject the ways you have known.

The Purification Principle honors the truth that each body is an ecosystem and each soul a unique expression of the same light. Yet there are universal laws at work. Laws of cleansing, flow, and renewal that every human can follow. These laws are not imposed by man but are the same laws that keep the tides in motion and the sap rising in spring.

To walk with The Purification Principle is to walk with these laws, to learn their language, and to let them work upon you. We begin to trust that under the layers of fatigue, craving, inflammation, grief, distraction, and numbness there is a self who is untouched, luminous, and free.

This book is an offering. A river map. A remembering. We will travel through the terrains of body, mind, and spirit, clearing what blocks the flow, restoring what feeds our vitality, and fortifying the channels so they remain unbroken. You will learn of plants that carry the memory of the sun, of practices that breathe wind into stagnant waters, and of ways to stand rooted in purity even as the world swirls with impurity around you.

The way ahead is not harsh. This is honest. When the last stone of interference is lifted from the riverbed of your being, you will see, as those who came before us saw, that purity is not a goal but is your nature.

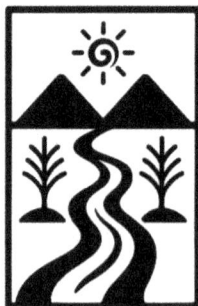

Chapter I: The Principle Defined

The Purification Principle begins with a simple truth: *what is pure needs no fixing.* The work is not to add more, but to remove what does not belong.

In the high mountains, far from roads, there is a spring that feeds a small meadow. The water emerges clear and cold from the rock, having passed through layers of earth and stone that have strained, polished, and blessed this source of sustenance. There is no requirement for a filter. The molecular structure is whole.

Your body, your mind, and your spirit, they are like that spring. Beneath the accumulation of years, beneath the sediments of choice and chance, beneath the silt of grief, stress, and environmental burden, you are clear. The Purification Principle is the remembering of this fact and the disciplined, gentle art of returning to this state.

There are three movements to this art:

1.) Removing Interference
2.) Restoring Flow
3.) Rebuilding Resilience.

Removing Interference

This is the clearing of the riverbed and lifting of stones and debris so the current can run without obstruction.

Interference comes in many forms:

• Physical toxins through food, water, air, and skin.

• Mental toxins of overstimulation, fear, and false narratives.

• Emotional toxins from unresolved wounds and shame.

• Subtle energetic residues from people and patterns.

In many indigenous traditions, cleansing was not occasional. This was woven into life. The people burned cedar, sage, or palo santo not to follow fashion, but because the smoke binds and carries away stagnation. The villagers fasted with the seasons to rest the organs and allowed inner fires to burn away the unnecessary. The healers prescribed sweat lodges and river immersions not as novelty, but as medicine to remind the body what freedom feels like.

Removing interference is not punishment. This is kindness, an act of hospitality toward your own inner guest, being the soul that chose to inhabit this body.

Restoring Flow

Once the obstructions are lifted, the river must be reminded of how to run. Flow is life. In the human being, flow is breath that moves without constriction, blood that circulates without stagnation, lymph that clears waste without sluggishness, and thoughts that pass like clouds without becoming storms.

Nature teaches this without a word. The forest does not hoard her rain; she lets each droplet submerge and seep and spill and cycle. The wind does not hold onto breath; the air moves from mountain to plain, reshaping both. Flow is how life distributes nourishment and removes waste.

We restore flow through breathwork, through movement that awakens the fascia and joints, through hydration that carries minerals into every cell, through plant-based nourishment that digests with ease, and through rest that lets the body repair. We restore flow by remembering the cycles. Sleeping in harmony with darkness, waking with light, and moving in rhythm with seasons rather than against them is aligning with higher harmonies.

Rebuilding Resilience

When the river runs clear and free, we tend the banks, so the flow does not flood or dry. Resilience is the capacity to meet challenges without collapse. This is the memory of wholeness that persists even under strain.

Resilience is built in the mitochondria, in the quiet work of enzymes, and in the fortification of the microbiome. This is built on the nervous system's ability to shift from fight to rest without getting stuck. We construct this ceaseless will in the spirit's trust that even in trial, the current carries us somewhere meaningful.

Our ancestors knew resilience was a form of wealth. They told stories not just to pass time, but to pass strength. These consisted of tales of endurance, winters survived, migrations completed, and healings against odds. Today, we rebuild resilience through whole foods, medicinal plants, light and movement, cultivating relationships that nourish instead of depleting, and through practices that anchor us in meaning.

The Principle as a Compass

The Purification Principle is not linear. Removing, restoring, and rebuilding are movements that are circular, like seasons. We are always clearing, reawakening flow, and fortifying the channels that hold what is sacred.

You may begin with a cleanse to remove interference, find that breathwork naturally restores your flow, and then strengthen your body with vibrant plants to build resilience. Or you may find that building resilience through nutrient-dense food gives you the strength to release deeper emotional toxins. There is no wrong place to begin, only the wrong assumption that you must wait.

In the esoteric schools, initiation is said to begin the moment you turn toward the light. The Purification Principle begins the moment you decide to become a clear vessel again. Not perfect, or untouchable, but clear.

The compass will point you back to your nature repeatedly. In time, the interference will fall away like old bark from a tree, revealing the living wood beneath. The flow will return like the spring thaw, unstoppable once begun. The resilience will become a forest root system under your feet, holding you steady in storms.

In the chapters ahead, we will walk this terrain together, naming the interferences, calling forth the flows, and cultivating resilience until this becomes your second nature. This is a return, not a race.

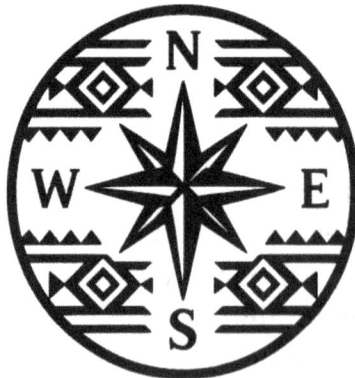

Chapter II: Removing Interference

Every river has stones. Some belong there, holding the banks steady and giving the water a place to sing. Others are fallen debris. Branches rotting, boulders from an upstream landslide, or silt from a careless crossing clogging the current and dulling the water's voice.

The body is no different. Some weight is necessary: *bones to anchor, minerals to conduct, and memory to guide.* Over time, though, we gather debris that does not serve us. We breathe in the fumes of cities, swallow the residues of chemicals, carry the stress of years, and absorb griefs we never name. Our river within grows sluggish, not because there is no recollection of how to flow, but because our fluids are carrying what was never meant to stay.

Removing interference is the first act of devotion in The Purification Principle. This is the offering of space back to the current.

The Four Realms of Interference

1.) Physical Interference: The Seen Stones

These are the toxins you can name and often measure: *pesticides in food, heavy metals in water, microplastics in the ocean and now in our blood, residues of pharmaceuticals lingering in tissues, and endocrine disruptors in plastics and perfumes.*

In the villages of the highlands, elders spoke of *"unfriendly guests"* in the body. Things that come to stay uninvited. They taught that one must seasonally *"sweep the house"* to keep such guests from making a home. This sweeping might be a fast of pure water, a few days of mono-meals like kitchari or papaya, or a week drinking only fresh-pressed juices from the land.

Plants that aid this clearing are the river's true allies:

• Cilantro and chlorella to bind heavy metals.
• Dandelion root to sweep the liver.
• Milk thistle to mend the hepatocytes after their labor.
• Burdock to filter the blood through the skin and kidneys.
• Lemon and ginger to cut mucus and enliven digestion.

Physical interference asks for honesty. Not punishment, or obsession, but a willingness to look at what we consume, breathe, and touch, and choose again.

2.) Mental Interference: The Tangled Currents

A clear river can become dangerous if the water loops back, trapped in an eddy. The mind works the same way. Thoughts that circle without resolution become stagnant pools, breeding restlessness and doubt.

The elders taught that words and images are food for the mind, and just as the body grows sick from polluted food, the mind sickens from polluted input. Today, we feed our minds with constant news, noise, and scrolling and wonder why our clarity dims.

Removing mental interference means cultivating sacred silence each day, even for a few minutes. This directs replacing hours of passive consumption with the living presence of the natural world. The wind in the pines, arc of a hawk's flight, and even the sound of your own breath.

Simple rituals help:

• Begin the morning without screens for the first hour.
• End the day with ten breaths counted like prayer beads.
• Speak less and listen more.
• Rest your mind in spaciousness, where clarity naturally gathers.

3.) Emotional Interference: The Mud of Memory

Rivers flood when they cannot absorb what comes; the banks give way and the waters cloud with mud. In the body, this flooding is the unprocessed emotional residuum of grief, anger, and fear that has nowhere to go.

In many indigenous traditions, grief is not a private burden but a communal song. The cry is offered to the fire, to the drum, and to the circle. This releases the emotion into the wider holding of the tribe and land. Without such release, emotions calcify, becoming stones in the heart's river. When we let the river carry the mud downstream, we find the waters lighten on their own.

To remove emotional interference:

• Name the feeling without judgment.
• Give breath and movement.
• Walk, dance, and sway until the tension softens.
• Offer the blockage to an element.
• Speak the obstacle to water.
• Burn the impedance in fire.
• Bury this burden in our earth.
• Let the wind carry away what does not belong.
• Seek counsel from those who know how to hold space.

4.) Energetic Interference: The Invisible Nets

Some stones you cannot see but can feel: *the heaviness after certain conversations, fatigue after walking through certain places, or the lingering of someone else's sorrow in your chest.*

Energy, like water, moves best when clean and unobstructed. Ancient ways knew this: *smudging with herbs, bathing in moving water, singing to break stagnant air, and drumming to realign the heartbeat of a space.*

You can clear energetic interference daily:

• Brush your body lightly from head to toe as though sweeping away dust.

• Spend time barefoot on soil or stone to discharge static and absorb the earth's current.

• Burn resins or herbs that speak to you, whether frankincense, copal, cedar, or sage, letting the smoke rise and old heaviness leave.

• Keep a stone or talisman that has been blessed in sunlight or river water, touching when you feel unmoored.

The First Clearing

In the early days of walking with The Purification Principle, begin gently. Choose one stone to lift from your river: *remove a processed food, replace a nightly scroll with a walk under stars, forgive one old wound, smudge your home at dawn.*

The river does not demand all her stones at once; she asks only that you begin the clearing. Each stone lifted lightens the current, and the lighter the current, the easier the path we have to find and free the next.

We begin here, with hands in the water, with the willingness to lift what no longer belongs, and with the knowing that beneath every stone lies the clarity we have been seeking all along.

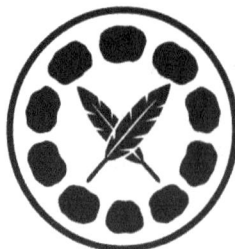

Chapter Three: Restoring Flow

A newly cleared river does not always remember her song. After years of sluggishness, the current must learn again how to dance around stones, how to braid waters, and how to feed the banks without drowning them. So too must the human body, mind, and spirit remember the art of movement once the obstructions have been lifted.

Flow is life's language. The tree speaks this when sap rises in spring. The ocean speaks of this continuation in the inhalation and exhalation of tides. Blood speaks fluidity in the quiet corridors of your veins. Breath speaks constancy each time oxygen enters as gift and leaves transformed as offering.

When flow is restored, the whole being hums in unison. Cells receive nutrients without resistance. Waste leaves without protest. Thoughts arrive, serve their purpose, and dissolve. Emotions move like weather, present but never permanent. Spirit moves through the vessel without catching on old snags.

The elders say: *stagnation is death; movement is life.* To restore flow, we look to the natural systems within us and around us.

Breath: First Current of the River

Before the first sip of water and first mouthful of food, breath is the original nourishment. The tide that moves through you twenty thousand times a day, shaping your chemistry with every rise and fall.

In many lineages, the breath is more than oxygen; this is referenced as prana, chi, and the unseen wind that carries life force. A stagnant breath is like a blocked tributary that chokes the downstream waters.

To restore the flow of breath:

• Begin each morning with conscious inhales and slow, complete exhales, as though sweeping the inner channels clean.

• Use cyclic breathing, four counts in, four counts out, to reset the nervous system during moments of mental stagnation.

• Practice deep belly breathing before meals, signaling safety to your body so digestion flows without tension.

Breath is the river's beginning. Clear the air and every other current will follow.

The Waters Within: Hydration as Ceremony

Flow demands water. Not merely the absence of thirst, but true cellular hydration, where every drop carries minerals into the tissues and waste out again.

Our ancestors drank from springs that carried the memory of stone, rain, and root. Today, much of what we call water has been stripped and sterilized, the structure and spirit dulled. To restore flow, we must give our bodies water that remembers how to nourish. When you drink, let this be a small ceremony as the return of the river to the river.

Practices to hydrate as the ancients might:

• Choose filtered water in glass that is restructured.

• Add a pinch of unrefined sea salt or a squeeze of lemon to awaken the water's conductivity.

• Drink upon waking, before food, to flush the night's stagnation.

• Sip steadily through the day rather than flooding the system all at once.

Movement: Stirring the Channels

Still water breeds algae; still limbs breed stagnation. Movement restores the microcurrents that keep blood, lymph, and energy in circulation. This is not the frantic motion of over-exercise, but the daily, rhythmic stirring that the body recognizes as joy. Movement is the stirring stick in the pot that keeps the contents from burning or settling.

To restore flow through movement:

• Walk upon the earth daily, allowing your spine to sway like the trunk of a young tree in wind.

• Use rebounding, shaking, or dancing to stimulate the lymph, the body's silent river of immunity.

• Stretch the fascia slowly, like drawing open a curtain to let light in.

• Move with the seasons: in winter, conserve with slow, strengthening work; in spring, let movement be playful and light; in summer, vigorous and open; in autumn, grounding and measured.

Rhythm: The Seasonal Pulse

Flow follows the cycles of the greater world. Nothing is random. The moon pulls the tides, the sun draws sap up the trunks, and the seasons turn the wheel of all living things. When our rhythms fall out of step with these cycles, stagnation seeps back into the river.

Indigenous calendars were less about marking days and more about marking flows — migrations, blooms, harvests, thaws. The Purification Principle asks us to return to this way of timekeeping.

To restore seasonal flow:

• Rise close to sunrise, sleep soon after dark, aligning your inner tides with light and shadow.

• Eat with the land's calendar. Cooling foods in summer, warming in winter, and transitional in spring and fall.

• Keep a practice that marks the turning points. Track solstice, the equinox, new moon, and full moon as moments to check the health of your flow.

Flow as Daily Devotion

Restoring flow is the ongoing choice to live like a river that refuses to be dammed. Some days, this will mean a long walk and a deep sweat. Other days, a quiet breath before bed and a glass of clean water in the morning. We emphasize the awareness, more than the effort, that keeps the channels open.

When breath moves without block, when water nourishes without pause, and when limbs stir and seasons are honored, flow becomes your default state. In flow, the body, mind, and spirit do what they have always known how to do. They carry life forward without holding on to what no longer belongs.

The river, once freed, does not ask permission to run. Neither should you.

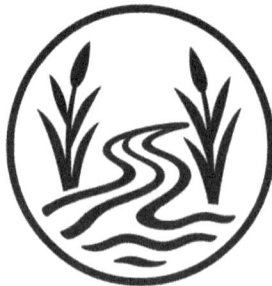

Chapter Four: Rebuilding Resilience

Once the stones are lifted from the riverbed and current moves freely again, the work turns to the tending of the banks. Without strong roots, a flood will carry them away. Without shade, the summer heat will dry the waters to a trickle. Flow alone is not enough. This fluid movement must be protected, nourished, and sustained.

Resilience is this protection. The quiet strength that allows the river to meet drought without disappearing, and to meet storm without breaking course.

In the human being, resilience is not built by avoiding challenge, but by engaging in ways that leave us stronger. This includes the cellular memory of survival, the spirit's ability to find meaning amid hardship, and the body's capacity to restore balance after strain.

The Roots Beneath the Water

Our ancestors knew that resilience begins in the smallest places. Even in the hidden work of roots. In the body, these roots are the mitochondria, the microbiome, the mineral reserves in the bones, and the adaptability of the nervous system. When these are strong, the whole being stands firm. When they are neglected, even a small wind can topple us.

Mitochondria are the tiny furnaces in your cells. They turn the food you eat into energy that fuels every thought, heartbeat, and movement. These furnaces are fed not only by calories, but by clean air, pure water, natural light, and plant compounds that repair and strengthen their walls.

The microbiome is the living forest inside you. Trillions of bacteria, fungi, and other microorganisms that digest your food, regulate your immune system, and even influence your mood. A diverse, thriving microbiome is like a resilient forest.

Feeding the Roots

To rebuild resilience, feed these foundations well:

• Eat the rainbow of plant foods to deliver the full spectrum of phytonutrients (see Plant Color Healing Guide).

• Include fermented foods like sauerkraut, kimchi, and coconut yogurt to seed beneficial microbes.

• Seek out adaptogens, plants like ashwagandha, rhodiola, holy basil, and reishi mushroom, which train the body to handle stress without exhaustion.

• Spend time in wild nature, letting your skin, lungs, and senses be touched by the microbiomes of forests, oceans, and meadows.

Plant Color Healing

Red

The color of heart-fire and circulation's song. Rich in lycopene and anthocyanins, these foods warm the blood, strengthen the heart, and quiet the low embers of inflammation.

Eat the hues of crimson and scarlet: ripe tomatoes, sun-kissed watermelon, wild strawberries, and sweet red bell peppers.

Orange

The light of sunset made edible. Infused with beta-carotene and bioflavonoids, these foods enhance your vision, awaken immune tides, and mend the skin's delicate weaves.

Turn to carrots, sweet potatoes, the dense flesh of pumpkin, and citrus that tastes of the sun.

Yellow

The golden lanterns of the plant kingdom. Bearing lutein and zeaxanthin, they guard the eyes, nourish the mind's clarity, and bring brightness to digestion.

Gather yellow squash, sunlit corn, fragrant pineapple, and the deep earth glow of turmeric.

Green

The color of renewal and the body's quiet cleansing. Chlorophyll and isothiocyanates run through them like a forest stream, washing, alkalizing, and strengthening the liver's steady labor.

Fill your basket with kale, spinach, broccoli, tender parsley, and the vital shoots of wheatgrass.

Blue/Purple

The night sky's wisdom made into food. Anthocyanins and resveratrol whisper to the brain, slow the aging clock, and keep the vessels supple.

Savor blueberries, blackberries, the deep crunch of purple cabbage, and the silk of roasted eggplant.

White/Tan

The cloaked healers of the plant realm. Allicin and polyphenols move quietly, dismantling invaders, fortifying immunity, and dismantling rogue cells before they take root.

Welcome burdock root, cauliflower, celery root, dragon fruit, and ginger into your daily ritual. To combat sickness, occasional garlic and leeks can be used medicinally.

The Nervous System's Riverbanks

Resilience lives in the nervous system's ability to shift between action and rest. Too much time in fight-or-flight mode erodes the banks, wearing down the spirit. Too much collapse and withdrawal let silt build up, dulling the current.

Indigenous and native peoples often built their days around rhythmic activities that naturally regulated the nervous system: *sunrise songs, midday rests, evening storytelling, and seasonal dances.* These rituals were more than culture; they were medicine, keeping the collective and individual nervous systems in balance.

When we return to these patterns, we invite the body into the timeless language of the earth. A language written in light and dark, movement and stillness, sound and silence. The nervous system, like a riverbank, cannot be endlessly battered without consequence. Restoration of our nerves must be built up with gentle deposits of safety and beauty. These deposits are made in moments of presence, in breath that reaches the belly, and in the simple act of lifting your eyes to the sky and remembering that you belong to something vast, steady, and benevolent.

You can tend your own riverbanks by:

• Practicing daily grounding by standing barefoot on earth, feeling the steadiness beneath you.

• Using breathwork to soften the heart rate after stress.

• Taking intentional pauses to witness beauty such as a bird's flight or the way sunlight moves on water.

• Ending the day with gratitude rituals, which shift the nervous system toward rest.

Strength Through Challenge

Resilience does not grow in the absence of challenge. A river becomes stronger when it has moved through flood and drought; its path deepens, its banks harden, its course becomes clear.

In our bodies and lives, this means meeting the small discomforts that prepare us for larger storms:

• Finishing a shower with a blast of cold to train the vascular system.

• Fasting occasionally to strengthen metabolic flexibility.

• Engaging in physical work builds functional strength rather than only aesthetics.

• Allowing moments of emotional vulnerability, trusting that openness does not break us but deepens our roots.

These acts, though simple, awaken ancient intelligence within. This is the same intelligence that guides the salmon upstream, that urges the seed to split the shell in darkness, and that carries the sap up the trunk before the frost has fully retreated. To choose challenge with awareness is to align yourself with the cosmic law of growth through contrast. We become, as all enduring things in nature are, shaped by the elements we have endured. We are polished by wind, tempered by fire, and strengthened by the press of stone and the pull of tide.

In the words of one Lakota elder: *"The willow survives the storm because he bends. The oak survives because she holds."* Resilience is knowing when to bend and when to hold.

31

Resilience as a Living Practice

When resilience is woven into daily life, purity can withstand the impurities of the world without being dimmed. You will still encounter toxins, grief, and strain, but they will pass through you like a brief storm over a deep river.

Rebuilding resilience is not about hardening against the world; this is about becoming so rooted, so nourished, and so aligned with your own flow that nothing foreign can stay for long. The wind may sway you, the flood may rise, but the core remains unbroken.

This is the resilience we cultivate in The Purification Principle: not brittle defense, but supple strength; not rigid purity that shatters under pressure, but living purity that adapts, heals, and continues.

When we live this way, we become like the rivers our ancestors drank from. We are clear, alive, and enduring.

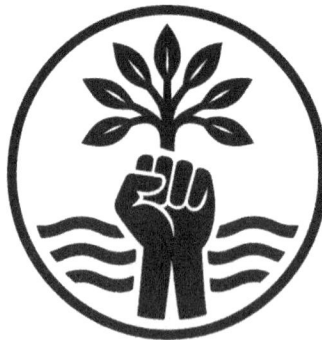

Chapter Five: The Purifier's Path

Once you have begun to remove the stones, restore the flow, and strengthen the banks, the question becomes: *How do I live this way, not as a project, but as a way of being?* The Purification Principle is not a seasonal cleanse or a temporary retreat from the world. This is a compass you carry every day, in every season, and under every sky.

The Purifier's Path is walked step by step. Sometimes slow, and sometimes swift, but always in the direction of greater clarity, greater vitality, and greater truth. We are stepping into alignment.

Daily Rituals: The Small Stones of the Path

A path is made by walking the direction daily. The practices you repeat, morning after morning, and evening after evening, are the stones that hold the way firm beneath your feet. They are invitations to step in as a clear vessel.

In the villages where the land was still the clock, life began with offerings. A pinch of cornmeal to the earth. A bowl of water poured at the base of a tree. A breath of smoke released toward the sky. These gestures were less about religion than about relationships. They served as reminders that we live in exchange with the world around us.

Your daily rituals may be as simple as:

• **Greeting the day with breath** — three slow inhales, three slow exhales, eyes open to the sky.
• **Drinking water as ceremony** — holding with both hands and offering thanks before swallowing.
• **Moving the body with intention** — stretching, walking, dancing, shaking off the night's stagnation.
• **Eating in stillness** — without screens or rush, chewing as though extracting the sun from each bite.

Seasonal Guidance: Walking with the Wheel of the Year

The Purifier's Path does not move in a straight line but in a circle, like the medicine wheels of indigenous traditions. Each season asks for a different way of tending to the self:

Spring: The Rising Sap

• Lighten the load.

• Favor raw greens, tender shoots, and cleansing herbs like nettle and dandelion.

• Move more, shed more, and let the flow quicken.

Summer: The Full Bloom

• Nourish with abundance.

• Eat colorful fruits and vegetables at their peak.

• Drink more water.

• Rest in the shade of the day and rise with the long light.

Autumn: The Gathering and Letting Go

• Harvest what is ripe. Not just food, but wisdom from the year's work.

• Eat grounding foods like squash and grains. Release what you cannot carry into winter.

Winter: The Deep Root

• Slow down.

• Favor warm, cooked foods, deep rest, and reflection.

• Strengthen resilience with medicinal plant broths and adaptogenic herbs.

• Tend the inner fire.

The Purifier's Mind

On this path, the mind is not an enemy but a river to be kept clear. This means guarding your intellectual intake as you would guard the source of your drinking water. Too much noise, too much fear, and too much comparison provide an environment for the waters to cloud.

Practice *mental fasting*: periods each day with no news, no social media, no artificial stimulation. Let silence be part of your nourishment. Feed the mind beauty, truth, and stories that strengthen your roots rather than erode them.

The Purifier's Heart

Purification without compassion becomes harsh. The Purifier's Path asks you to keep the heart soft, even as you clear away what does not belong.

This may mean forgiving yourself for years of neglect, forgiving others for harm, and forgiving the world for being imperfect. The heart that forgives is not naive but free.

Tend to your relationships. Speak honestly. Listen deeply. Offer help when you can and accept help when offered to you. Purity grows fastest in soil shared with others.

The Purifier's Spirit

The spirit thrives on connection. To the land, to the unseen, and to the mystery that holds us all. You may find this connection in prayer, meditation, time in the wilderness, or in creative work that brings you into timelessness.

Make a place in your home that is an altar. Not necessarily of religion, but of remembrance. A candle, a stone, a feather, or a cup of water. Any objects that remind you of your place in the great weave. Visit this sacred space daily. Offer something: *a word, a breath, a piece of fruit, a song.*

Walking On

The Purifier's Path is not about arriving at a final destination where you are "pure" forever. It is about living in a way where interference is addressed as it arises, flow is restored before stagnation takes hold, and resilience is nourished through the seasons.

There will be days when you stumble — days when you eat what dulls you, speak what clouds you, ignore what would renew you. These are not failures; they are reminders to return to the path. The river finds its way back to the sea no matter how many times it bends.

Walk this path with patience. Walk it with reverence. Walk it knowing that every step in alignment, no matter how small, is a step toward the clear water you were born from and will return to.

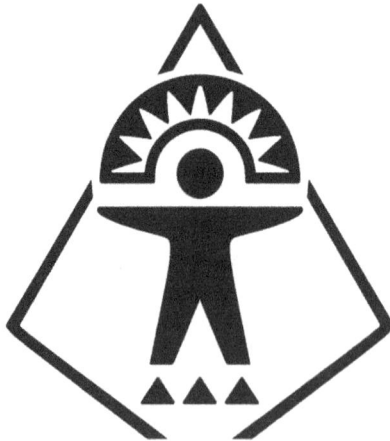

Chapter Six: The Purifier's Kitchen

The kitchen is not just a place of preparation; this is a temple of transformation. Here, the alchemy of earth, water, fire, and air turns seeds into sustenance, leaves into medicine, and roots into strength. Every meal is a ceremony and each ingredient a messenger carrying the story of soil.

For those walking The Purification Principle, the kitchen is where theory becomes life. Where the removal of interference, the restoration of flow, and the rebuilding of resilience are all practiced in the language of food.

Food as Living Medicine

The elders remind us: *If food does not rot, this cannot feed life.* Food that is alive, fresh, vibrant, and seasonal, carries the lifeforce of the sun, the rain, and the soil. Food that is dead, refined, or stripped of original form carries the shadow of convenience but not the essence of nourishment.

In indigenous foodways, there was no separation between food and medicine. The bitter greens of spring were not just for flavor. They woke the liver from winter rest. The roots of autumn steadied the body for the cold months ahead. Every color, texture, and taste aligned to the body's rhythm.

To eat as a purifier is to choose foods that carry no residue of harm. These are comprised of plant-sourced foods grown without poison, prepared with care, and eaten with awareness. To prepare food in this way is to enter relationships. Each knife stroke, stir of the pot, and moment of waiting as flavors marry, becomes a silent vow to honor both body and Earth. In this space, the kitchen becomes a sanctuary where nourishment is infused not only with nutrients, but with intention. Here, the act of eating is communion, a returning of gratitude to the soil, the seed, the water, and the unseen hands that allowed for this meal.

Plant Color Healing

As we introduced in chapter four, every color in the plant kingdom is an invitation to a particular kind of healing. When you fill your plate with many colors, you weave a spectrum of protection and renewal into your cells. We want our kitchen to be bright, colorful, vibrant and filled with radiance. We eat with the same diversity as the wild meadow, where each shade has purpose.

The goal is to gather an array of pigment-rich, antioxidant-dense foods for preparing juices, meals and smoothies for optimal nourishment.

Here are some colorful foods we recommend for your home:

Red: Lycopene and anthocyanins for heart and circulation: blood oranges, cherries, cranberries, pitaya, pomegranates, red bell peppers, strawberries, and watermelon.

Orange: Beta-carotene and bioflavonoids for eyes, immunity, and skin: apricots, cantaloupe, carrots, mango, orange citrus, papaya, persimmons, pumpkin, and sweet potato.

Yellow: Lutein and zeaxanthin for vision, brain clarity, and digestion: corn (raw & non-GMO), golden beets, lemon, passionfruit, peppers, pineapple, and turmeric.

Green: Chlorophyll and isothiocyanates for detox and liver health: arugula, asparagus, broccolini, cilantro, collards, kale, parsley, spinach, and wheatgrass.

Blue/Purple: Anthocyanins and resveratrol for longevity, brain, and blood vessels: acai, blackberries, blueberries, currants, figs, grapes, purple cabbage, and purple carrots.

White/Tan: Allicin and polyphenols for immunity, antimicrobial defense, and cancer prevention: cauliflower, coconut, ginger, parsnips, sunchokes, and white beans.

The Purifier's Pantry

A kitchen in alignment with the Purification Principle will be simple, but not sparse; and abundant but not cluttered. What you do *not* keep is equally important. Foods that clog the flow, whether ultra-processed items, refined sugars, oils stripped of their vitality, or animal products heavy with toxins, are simply not part of the temple.

To open such a pantry is to step into a sanctuary. Each jar and basket whispers of soil and sun, each spice carries the memory of distant fields, each tea leaf hums with the vibration of rain. A pantry kept in this way reminds you daily of your covenant with life. This is an altar of intention, where every item has a purpose and every meal begins long before the first bite.

Stock your home with what feeds life:

• **Fresh vegetables and fruits** — organic, seasonal, and ideally local.

• **Herbs and spices** — basil, cayenne, cilantro, cardamom, chili powder, cinnamon, coriander, cumin, dill, oregano, paprika, rosemary, sage, and turmeric.

• **Fermented foods** — sauerkraut, kimchi, coconut yogurt, miso, kefir from plant milks.

• **Seeds and nuts** — almonds, chia, flax, hemp, pecans, pistachios, pumpkin seeds, and walnuts.

• **Pseudograins and legumes** — adzuki beans, amaranth, black beans, black eye peas, lentils, millet, and mung beans.

• **Healing teas** — chamomile, ginger, gynostemia, hibiscus, nettles, and rooibos.

• **Pure water** — filtered, reverse-osmosis, then structured if possible, and always in glass not plastic.

Rituals of Preparation

How you prepare food is as much a part of the medicinal effect as what you prepare. In many cultures, cooking is accompanied by song, prayer, or gratitude. The hands that cook transfer their state of being into the meal.

Before cooking:

• Wash your hands in cool water, imagining the day's residue flowing off.

• Take a breath to center yourself.

• Give thanks to the plant, the land, and the unseen forces that brought the food into your hands.

While cooking:

• Keep the space uncluttered so the work feels sacred.
• Use tools and vessels that you enjoy touching and seeing.
• Move without rushing, letting the process be nourishing.

Cooking in this way is a ceremony of union. The plant offers sustenance, you offer your intention, and together something greater is born. The flavors deepen when gratitude is present, the aromas carry farther when the heart is open, and the meal becomes not just sustenance, but blessing. In this way, food ceases to be a commodity and becomes a dialogue between human and earth, between matter and spirit.

When the food is shared, the medicine is multiplied. A simple bowl of lentils, prepared with reverence, carries more life than a banquet cooked in haste. Every person who eats partakes not only of the nutrients but of the care infused in the preparation. The ritual stretches beyond your kitchen into the bodies and hearts of those you feed, weaving them into the same river of purity you yourself are walking.

The Purifier's Plate

A plate in harmony with The Purification Principle is vibrant, balanced, and easy for the body to process.

Think of your plate as a medicine wheel:

• Half is covered with raw or steamed organic vegetables of many colors.
• A quarter is filled with pseudograins or legumes for grounding.
• A quarter consists of healthy fats and proteins from seeds, nuts, and plant-based sources.

Season generously with herbs, citrus, and spices. Flavor is a part of vitality that awakens digestion and brings joy to the act of eating.

Eating as Prayer

In the Purifier's Kitchen, eating is never mindless. Sit down. Place your feet on the floor. Smell the food before taking a bite. Chew slowly, until the food is no longer distinct in texture. This is how your body extracts the full gift from every plant, every spice, every drop of water.

The kitchen is the heart of the home, and for the purifier, is the place where the river is fed daily. Here, you choose whether to cloud the waters or keep them clear. Each choice and every meal is a step deeper into the current of life that has always been waiting to carry you.

The elders say: *When you eat with gratitude, you feed more than the body; you feed the spirit.*

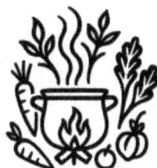

Chapter Seven: The Purifier's Medicine Chest

Every village, homestead, and traveling caravan once had a place where remedies were kept. Sometimes this was a carved wooden box, sometimes a clay jar sealed with wax, and sometimes simply a patch of earth outside the door where certain plants grew. This was the medicine chest. Not a sterile cabinet of pills, but a living collection of allies.

The Purifier's Medicine Chest is both literal and symbolic. The shelf of teas and tinctures in your kitchen, the pouch of dried herbs in your travel bag, and the bundle of cedar on your altar. This is also the collection of practices, memories, and rituals you turn to when the flow falters, the river clouds, or the banks begin to crumble.

The Philosophy of Plant Allies

In the old ways, plants were not *"supplements"* or *"commodities."* They were kin. Each had a spirit, a temperament, and a gift. The healer's art was not to dominate the plant, but to listen. To match the nature with the needs of the one seeking healing.

This is the first rule of the Purifier's Medicine Chest: *know your allies not just by name, but by character.* Ginger is the warming friend who stirs the blood when sluggish. Nettle is the quiet nurse who rebuilds what has been depleted. Tulsi is the holy one who calms the stormed mind without dulling any brightness.

Foundational Allies for the Purifier

Nettle (Urtica dioica)

• Mineral-rich and deeply nourishing, nettle feeds the blood, strengthens bones, and restores vitality after cleansing.

• Drink as an infusion, steeped for hours, for maximum strength.

Dandelion Root (Taraxacum officinale)

• The humble digger. Clears the liver, stimulates digestion, and encourages the release of old waste.

• Roast lightly for a coffee-like drink that heals instead of harms.

Milk Thistle (Silybum marianum)

• A guardian for the liver's cells, repairing and protecting after chemical or environmental stress.

• Take as a tincture or capsule, especially during detox phases.

Ginger (Zingiber officinale)

• The fire-bringer. Warms the body, stimulates circulation, and aids in breaking down stagnation in digestion.

• Use fresh in teas, juices, and meals.

Turmeric (Curcuma longa)

• The golden root of resilience. Anti-inflammatory, antioxidant, and cleansing to the blood.

• Combine with black pepper to awaken its full potency.

Cilantro & Chlorella

• A partnership for pulling heavy metals from tissues.

• Use cilantro fresh in meals, chlorella as a powder or tablet, but always ensure proper elimination channels are open.

Tulsi (Holy Basil, Ocimum sanctum)

• The sacred balancer. Calms the nervous system while sharpening mental clarity.

• Drink as a daily tea to harmonize mind, body, and spirit.

Reishi Mushroom (Ganoderma lucidum)

• The ancient tree healer. Builds immunity, deepens rest, and strengthens the body's adaptive capacity.

• Best taken as a long-brewed tea or quality extract.

Chilcuague (Heliopsis longipes)

• Known as the *golden root of the Aztecs*, chilcuague has been used for centuries as a sacred purifier of mouth, stomach, and blood.

• A spray or tincture of this fiery root awakens the salivary glands, cleanses the oral microbiome, and stirs the immune system into sharpness.

Black Salve

• A medicine carried quietly through generations, black salve is a drawing remedy, applied externally to pull toxins, infections, or growths toward the surface.

• Must be used with wisdom, guidance, and respect. When honored properly, this salve becomes a potent ally for the skin, calling out what does not belong and encouraging the body's own defenses to rise and release.

The Energetic Medicine Chest

Not all medicine grows from soil. Some is carried in smoke, song, and stone.

• **Cedar** — Clears heavy or stagnant energy from spaces and the self. Burn in the morning to reset a home.
• **Copal Resin** — Sacred to Mesoamerican peoples, copal lifts prayers and purifies the air.
• **Sage** — For clearing the unseen residue of conflict or grief; use with respect and intention.
• **Sea Salt** — A universal purifier; dissolve in bathwater or sprinkle in thresholds to cleanse and protect.
• **Crystals and Stones** — Black tourmaline for grounding, clear quartz for amplification, amethyst for spiritual clarity.

How to Work with the Medicine Chest

1. Build Slowly

Do not rush to collect everything at once. Begin with one or two allies and learn them deeply. Their taste, their effect, and their season of strength.

2. Store with Respect

Keep herbs in glass jars away from heat and light. Label them with their name, date, and where they were sourced.

3. Work Seasonally

In spring, favor bitters and greens. In summer, cooling herbs and hydration. In autumn, roots and adaptogens. In winter, warming spices and immune tonics.

4. Make the Medicine

Whenever possible, prepare your own infusions, decoctions, and salves. The act of making is part of the healing. Your intention infuses the remedy.

The Medicine Chest as Relationship

The Purifier's Medicine Chest changes with your needs, the seasons, and your own growth. Sometimes the inside is filled with strong tonics for deep cleansing. Other times there are simply gentle teas for quiet maintenance.

Remember: *the medicine chest is not about dependency.* These allies are not crutches, but companions on the path. Their purpose is to support your body's own wisdom.

When you keep such a chest that is living, respectful, and intentional, you are no longer at the mercy of every passing sickness or imbalance. You have the knowledge, the tools, and the relationships to meet what comes with grace. You have, in your own home, the same kind of quiet, steadying presence that healers once carried from village to village, knowing that health is not a product, but a relationship with life itself.

In this way, the medicine chest becomes not just a store of remedies, but a mirror of your own resilience. A reflection of the rivers, forests, and fields that live within you.

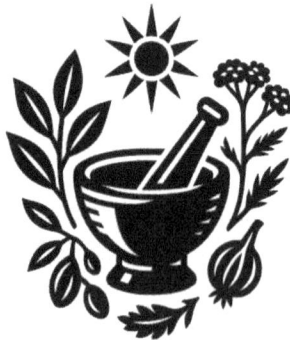

Chapter Eight: The Purifier's Practices

The Purification Principle is not sustained by theory alone. This is kept alive by what we *do*, and by the ways we meet each day and season.

Practices are examples of how we remind the body of our design, the mind of our clarity, and the spirit of our freedom. Without them, purity fades under the constant tide of interference. With them, purity is the natural state we return to repeatedly.

In the old ways, these practices were not called *"wellness routines"* or *"biohacks."* They were simply the ways of living, woven into the rhythm of sunrise and sunset, the migrations of animals, and the flowering of plants. The Purifier's Practices are our return to those rhythms, adapted to the world we live in now.

To practice is to remember. Each gesture, whether a breath, a sip of clean water, or a walk among trees, is a thread tying us back to the original design. These threads, woven day after day, become a fabric strong enough to hold us steady when the world pulls us toward forgetfulness. In this way, practice is less about discipline and more about devotion, a daily choosing of what we will align ourselves with: *interference or flow.*

So, the purifier emerges as an artist of rhythm. The body becomes the drum, the breath is the flute, and the seasons are the great orchestra. Every act of preparation, all moments of stillness, and each cleansing ritual is a note played in harmony with the larger song of life. When we practice, we step into that song, not as listeners alone, but as participants shaping the music.

Daily Practices: The Steady Current

These are the small acts that, done each day, keep the water from clouding. They do not need to be elaborate. Their power comes from their constancy.

1. Morning Breath Awakening

Before food, before screens, and even before speaking, take three slow breaths, deep into the belly, and release slowly, out through the mouth. Inhale clarity, exhale yesterday. If possible, do this facing the rising sun.

2. Hydration as Ritual

A glass of pure, mineral-rich water upon waking. Hold this in both hands. Offer thanks to the source, then drink slowly, imagining the liquid sustenance washing your cells like rain.

3. Movement to Stir the River

This need not be a workout; this is simply the stirring of circulation and lymph. This can be stretching, shaking, rebounding, walking barefoot in the yard, or slow yoga flow.

4. Plant-Based, Color-Full Meals

At least two meals each day filled with a variety of plant colors. Red for the heart, green for the liver, purple for the brain, and yellow for digestion. Each color is a note in the song of your healing.

5. Sunset Release

As the day closes, take a few moments to let go of what you need not carry into the night. This can be journaling, a short prayer, burning a slip of paper, or a slow exhale under the changing sky.

Weekly Practices: The Deep Rinse

Some cleansing requires a little more time and space. Once a week, offer yourself a deeper practice that sweeps through the whole system.

1. Nature Immersion

• At least once a week, spend one uninterrupted hour in nature with no agenda and no phone. Just be with the living world letting the natural flow recalibrate your own.

2. Extended Breathwork Session

• Choose a practice like circular breathing, box breathing, or alternate nostril breathing for 15–30 minutes. These patterns reset the nervous system and clear stagnant energy.

3. Herbal Bath or Sauna

• Soak with Epsom salts and herbs like lavender, rosemary, or chamomile, or sweat in a sauna, imagining each bead of sweat as a stone leaving your river.

4. Simplified Eating Window

• Once a week, condense your eating window to 6–8 hours, giving your digestion time to rest and your cells a chance to repair. Drink plenty of water and herbal tea during the fast.

5. Digital Silence

• Once a week, step away from screens and devices for a set period, perhaps a morning, an evening, or a full day if possible. This silence is not only for the eyes, but for the mind and spirit. Let the nervous system unclench from the constant stream of images and information. This is a fasting of the senses, a clearing of invisible clutter, and a way of remembering that your life is not contained in pixels but in breath, presence, and the living world around you.

Seasonal Practices: Walking with the Wheel

The earth changes, and so must our purification. Seasonal shifts offer natural checkpoints for deeper work.

Spring: Clearing the Winter Weight

• Favor greens, sprouts, and bitter herbs.

• Increase movement; let your body mirror the quickening of the earth.

• A 3–7 day gentle cleanse of juices, broths, and light salads.

Summer: Flow and Expansion

• Hydrate deeply with fruits like watermelon, cucumber, and berries.

• Spend more time outdoors, absorbing sunlight wisely.

• Engage in playful, joyful movement — swimming, hiking, dancing.

Autumn: Grounding and Release

• Shift to warming foods: squash, root vegetables, and pseudograins.

• Let go of excess, in possessions, habits, or relationships.

• Offer gratitude rituals for the year's harvest.

Winter: Deep Rest and Fortification

• Emphasize consciously cooked foods, soups, and adaptogens like reishi, ashwagandha, and astragalus.

• Sleep more and slow your pace. Reflect on the year's learnings.

• Gentle, inward practices: *meditation, journaling, and storytelling.*

The Spirit of Practice

The Purifier's Practices are not meant to be rigid demands. They are living invitations. Ways to keep your inner waters moving, channels open, and roots deep. Some days, you may do them all. Other days, only one or two. The important thing is not the number, but the remembering.

As one Diné elder once said: *"Our ceremonies are not for the gods. They are for us, so we do not forget the way home."*

Each practice is a small ceremony, bringing you home to your own clear nature. Do them long enough, and they cease to be *"practices"* at all. They become your way of being.

When practice ripens into way-of-being, the line between sacred and ordinary dissolves. Washing a bowl becomes as holy as prayer. Walking to the market carries the same weight as walking to the temple. Every act, no matter how small, becomes an echo of the river's song, reminding you that purity is not something you visit for a time, but the ground you stand on and the current that carries you, always.

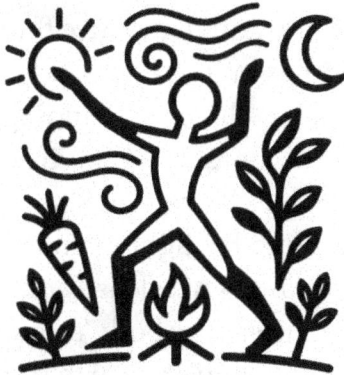

Chapter Nine: The Seasons of Purification

The earth does not cleanse herself in the same way every month. She turns, tilts, leans closer to the sun, then away. She floods and dries, blooms and sleeps. To live in purity is to move with her and to let your own river swell and rest in rhythm with the larger waters.

Purification, when guided by the seasons, becomes effortless. Each time of year holds unique medicine, and an invitation to clear, to nourish, and to renew.

In the spring, the earth reminds us that newness begins with shedding. Snow melts, rivers overflow, trees push out what has been stored in their roots. The body too longs for this clearing. A chance to lighten, to stir, and to flush away the heaviness of winter. To ignore this call is to move against the current; to heed is to ride with the season's tide of renewal.

Summer teaches abundance, but also the discipline of balance. The sun offers fire and energy in full measure, yet demands hydration, shade, and rhythm in return. Just as crops must be watered to bear fruit without burning in the heat, so must the body be cooled, replenished, and moved with respect for the intensity of the season. Summer is a time to both celebrate vitality and to practice the art of temperance.

Autumn and winter invite deeper lessons. The fall winds scatter what no longer clings, reminding us to let go, to harvest wisdom and compost what has reached an end. Winter, in her stillness, asks us to rest and rebuild, to honor the dark as fertile ground for light's return.

Together, these seasons of release and restoration are not endings, but sacred pauses. The body's way of conserving, the spirit's way of listening, and the earth's way of teaching us that death and rebirth are never separate, only different sides of the same turning wheel.

Spring: The Rising Sap

Spring is the season of upward movement. The frozen rivers break, the sap climbs the trees, and the soil loosens for new roots. In the body, this is the time to shake off the heaviness of winter and to wake the blood, lighten digestion, and sweep the channels clear.

Foods:

• Asparagus, dandelion leaves, fresh greens, nettles, radishes, and sprouts.

• Light fruits like berries and citrus.

•The first edible flowers such as calendula, dandelion, and violet blossoms.

Practices:

• Begin the day with lemon water to wake the liver.

• Include bitters daily, such as arugula, dandelion, and endive, to stimulate detox pathways.

• Move more: dancing, rebounding, stretching, and walking.

• Spring cleanse: 3–7 days of broths, herbal teas, juices, and salads.

Ritual:

At the equinox, write down what you are ready to grow and plant this with a seed. Let the earth hold your intention as the season unfolds.

Summer: The Full Bloom

Summer is expansion. The sun stands high, rivers run fast, and fruits swell with sweetness. The body's task is to maintain hydration, protect the heart from overheat, and flow with the abundance without becoming overindulgent.

Foods:

• High-water fruits such as cucumber, grapes, stone fruits, and watermelon.

• Cooling vegetables like celery, lettuce, and zucchini.

• Fresh herbs including basil, cilantro, dill, mint, parsley, and sage.

Practices:

• Begin mornings with hydrating fruits.

• Drink infusions of hibiscus, mint, and rose to cool the blood.

• Take movement outdoors by implementing barefoot walking, hiking, running, and swimming.

• Avoid heavy, greasy foods that overburden digestion in heat.

Ritual:

On the summer solstice, spend time in water, whether in a lake, river, sea, or bathing, offering gratitude for all that has come into bloom in your life.

Autumn: The Gathering & Letting Go

Autumn is the season of harvest and release. Trees draw sap down to their roots. Leaves fall. The air sharpens. In the body, this is the time to strengthen immunity, ground the energy, and let go of what will not serve through the winter.

Foods:

• Root vegetables such as beets, carrots, and sweet potatoes.

• Apples, pears, persimmons, pomegranate, pumpkin, and squash.

• Warming spices like cardamom, cinnamon, ginger, and turmeric.

Practices:

• Shift to warmer, cooked foods to prepare digestion for colder months.

• Eat fermented vegetables daily to support the microbiome.

• Begin gentle immune tonics such as astragalus, elderberry, and reishi.

• Release excess commitments, emotional burdens, and possessions.

Ritual:

At the autumn equinox, write down what you are ready to release, then burn or bury this burden, letting the land compost what remains into new life.

Winter: The Deep Root

Winter is the season of stillness. Rivers slow beneath ice. Seeds sleep in the dark soil. The body's work is to rest, rebuild, and conserve energy while keeping the inner fire alive.

Foods:

• Warm soups, stews, and veggie broths.

• Pseudograins like amaranth, buckwheat, and millet.

• Nuts, seeds, and dried fruits.

• Adaptogenic herbs including ashwagandha, chaga, and maca.

Practices:

• Sleep longer and rise later when possible.

• Practice gentle, grounding movement like yin yoga, qigong, or slow walks.

• Use warming spices like black pepper, cayenne, cloves, and ginger to stoke circulation.

• Reflect on the year: journal, meditate, and tell stories.

Ritual:

At the winter solstice, light a single candle in the darkness. Name aloud the inner fires you will tend until the sun returns.

The Circle Turns

When we live with the seasons, purification ceases to feel like a chore. The release becomes a dance. We feel light and quick in spring, full and flowing in summer, grounded and deliberate in autumn, and still and deep in winter.

In indigenous traditions across the world, the circle of the year was a teacher, not simply a calendar. The lessons were the same each year, yet they always met the people differently, depending on what they were carrying, what they had learned, and what they still needed to let go of.

Walking with this wheel, you find that purity is not a one-time achievement. This is a relationship with the living earth. A promise to tend your own river as she tends hers, in every season, for as long as you walk here.

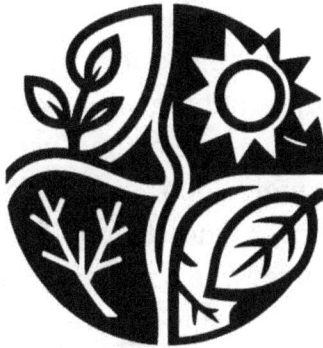

Chapter Ten: Advanced Purification Practices

There comes a time in the journey when the river is running clear, yet the purifier senses there are still hidden sediments deep in the bends, clinging to the roots, and sleeping beneath the sand. These are the places where the everyday practices cannot fully reach.

Advanced purification is for those who have already lightened their load, restored their flow, and built resilience, and now seek to refine by clearing the deepest channels, and awakening the subtlest currents. These practices draw from both ancient ceremonies and modern innovation, reminding us that purity is timeless, yet always evolving. The sweat lodge and the cold plunge, the fasting fire vigil and the hyperbaric chamber, the frog's purgative secretion and the hum of bioelectric frequency all are tools of the same principle. They meet us at different layers of being, entering where the gentler practices cannot yet penetrate.

To walk this path requires courage, for advanced purification often confronts us with what has been buried longest. The purge may be sudden, the visions unrelenting, and the release unlike anything we have known. In the very intensity, though, lies the medicine. Just as the river carves canyons deeper through flood, so too do these experiences carve us wider, stronger, and clearer. They are not meant to harm, but to strip away the final disguises of interference, bringing to the surface what is long hidden in shadow.

Here, discernment becomes the purifier's shield. Not every tool is meant for every person, nor at every stage of the journey. Some medicines demand readiness of spirit, others require physical preparation, and all are encouraged to include a circle of support and wise guidance.

Advanced practices are not badges to collect, but thresholds to cross with reverence. The body will speak when time, the dreams will signal, and the inner voice will whisper: *Now you are ready.*

In that readiness, the purifier learns that the great river of life holds many tributaries. Ancient songs, indigenous rituals, cutting-edge science, and modern technology can all serve as pathways back into flow. When chosen with integrity, they do not compete, they conspire together. They remind us that the pursuit of purity is not about clinging to tradition or novelty alone, but about weaving the wisdom of both into a practice that touches every hidden stone.

Ceremonial Purifications

Kambo: The Jungle's Warrior Medicine

Kambo is the secretion of the Amazonian, bicolor phyllomedusa tree frog, applied to small points on the skin in a sacred, guided ceremony. This is a physical, purgative medicine, that is not psychoactive and works swiftly to purge toxins from the lymphatic system, awaken the immune defenses, and clear emotional heaviness. At SoulSpire, Kambo is held in reverence, and guided with preparation, intention, and integration as a reset for the body and cleansing for the spirit.

Sacred Sweat: Heat as Purifier

From the Lakota Inipi to Finnish saunas, sweat has always been a universal cleansing method. In advanced practice, extended heat combined with cold immersion becomes an initiation, expanding circulation, expelling toxins through the skin, and training the nervous system to remain calm in extremes.

Internal Cleansing

Colon Hydrotherapy: The River's Channel

The health of the entire body is anchored in the cleanliness of the colon. This is the river's channel where waste is meant to leave swiftly, and water is intended to run clear. When the colon is sluggish or clogged, every upstream current suffers. Toxins recirculate, inflammation builds, the immune system falters, and vitality wanes.

Colon hydrotherapy is the direct washing of this channel; a modern extension of practices found in nearly every ancient culture. In Egypt, reeds were used to cleanse with water. In Ayurveda, Basti therapies were central to seasonal renewal. Indigenous healers taught that the bowels must be kept moving daily if the spirit was to remain light.

At SoulSpire, colon hydrotherapy is honored as one of the most foundational practices, reminding us that without a clear channel, no other purification can flow efficiently.

Enema Therapies: Targeted Streams of Healing

Where colon hydrotherapy is a broad cleansing of the whole channel, enemas are like tributaries. These are targeted streams carrying specific medicines into the river. Enema therapies have long been revered not only for clearing, but for delivering concentrated healing directly to the colon, where absorption is rapid and potent.

Organic coffee enemas stimulate the liver to release bile and toxins, opening one of the body's most powerful detox gates. Herbal enemas with chamomile, aloe, garlic, or chlorophyll can soothe inflammation, fight pathogens, and restore balance to the intestinal terrain. Mineral or probiotic enemas can replenish what has been lost, reseeding vitality into the deepest soil of the gut.

Oxygen Technologies

Ozone Therapy: The Oxygen Surge

Ozone is oxygen in an activated form, containing three atoms instead of two, and is one of nature's most potent antimicrobials. This treatment clears viral, bacterial, and fungal burdens while oxygenating tissues deeply. In the purifier's journey, ozone therapy can target hidden infections and restore cellular vitality in ways other methods cannot.

Hyperbaric Oxygen: The Deep Saturation

In hyperbaric oxygen therapy (HBOT), the body is bathed in pressurized oxygen, which dissolves into plasma and reaches tissues that normal breathing cannot touch. This accelerates healing, reduces inflammation, and enhances brain function. At SoulSpire, HBOT is offered as both a recovery tool and longevity practice. A way to feed dormant parts of the river.

Vibrational & Frequency Healing

BioCharger: Light, Frequency, and Voltage

The BioCharger combines pulsed electromagnetic fields, frequency therapy, light spectrum exposure, and voltage to re-energize cells. Think of standing in a modern-day sun, designed to awaken the body's own repair systems.

Rife Therapy: The Song of the Cells

Every organism has a resonant frequency. Rife technology uses specific sound and light frequencies to target pathogens and restore cellular harmony. Where conventional methods might kill indiscriminately, Rife aims to disrupt only what does not belong, leaving the body's beneficial systems untouched.

PEMF: The Cellular Pulse

Pulsed Electromagnetic Field therapy (PEMF) works by sending rhythmic waves of energy through the body, gently recharging the electrical potential of each cell. Every cell is like a small battery, and over time, stress, toxicity, and stagnation drain the charge. When the current falls too low, the body struggles to repair, communicate, and defend.

PEMF reawakens these microcurrents, restoring the natural voltage that drives cellular metabolism. Blood flow improves, oxygen delivery increases, and tissues are repaired more efficiently. Many describe the sensation as attunement. A reminder of the body's original frequency, harmonized again with the earth's magnetic field.

At SoulSpire, PEMF is offered as a bridge between deep rest and active recovery. For the purifier, this is a way of remembering that health is electrical as much as chemical, and that when the body's inner circuitry is restored, the river of life can move unimpeded through every channel.

Sound and Vibration Baths

From Tibetan singing bowls to modern vibroacoustic therapy, sound has the power to move what is stuck in the body's waters. Vibrational healing is powerful for emotional debris from grief, trauma, and old fear stored in the tissues.

When immersed in sound, the body becomes an instrument. The waters resonate with each tone and tissues loosen where frequency meets resistance. The drumbeat grounds the heartbeat, the bowl hum softens the mind's grip, and the chant or hum opens the chest until breath and spirit move freely again. In this way, sound does not merely soothe; but reorganizes, tuning the inner rivers back into harmony with the larger music of creation.

Layering These Practices

Advanced purification often works best when modalities are combined. At SoulSpire, there are not random offerings. The services are woven into personalized protocols, layered in the correct sequence so the body is ready for each step.

• Ozone to clear microbial and toxic burdens.

• Hyperbaric oxygen to super-saturate tissues with lifeforce.

• Kambo to purge the lymph and emotional body.

• BioCharger to re-energize cells and restore coherence.

• Rife therapy to fine-tune the internal environment.

• Colon hydrotherapy to cleanse the intestinal channel and lighten the body's overall burden.

• Sweating and contrast therapy to move waste and train resilience.

Layering purification is an art, not a checklist. Each modality has a distinct tone, rhythm, and depth of reach. When arranged with wisdom, they create a symphony. One practice prepares the terrain for the next, each building upon the other like instruments joining a song.

Ozone clears what clogs the tissues so that hyperbaric oxygen can saturate more deeply. Kambo purges emotional and lymphatic burdens, making way for frequency therapies like Rife or the BioCharger to resonate without obstruction. Colon hydrotherapy opens the body's root channel, ensuring waste is released rather than recirculated, amplifying the effectiveness of every other practice. Contrast therapy then moves the stirred debris out of the system, sealing the work with resilience. In this way, the body is never overwhelmed.

At SoulSpire, layering is approached like weaving a basket: *every strand strengthens the others, and the design is adapted to the unique shape of each person's river.* No two protocols are identical, because no two bodies carry the same stones or flow in the same direction. What remains constant is the principle to prepare, energize, and restore, until the current runs not only clean, but strong enough to carry the soul where one longs to go.

Walking with Respect

Advanced purification is not about doing more for the sake of more. This is about precision, knowing the river well enough to see where she runs heavy, and choosing the right tool for that bend. This requires physical, mental, and spiritual preparation and demands integration afterward. A deep purge without follow-up nourishment is like dredging a river but leaving the banks bare.

In indigenous teaching, the deeper the medicine, the more careful the ceremony. The same is true here. These tools are powerful not because they are extreme, but because they reach where few others can.

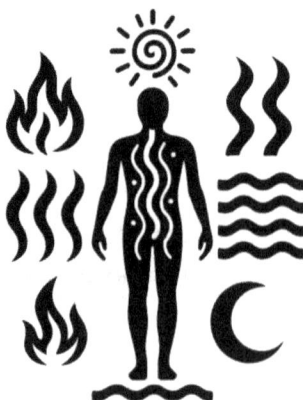

Chapter Eleven: Living Purity in an Impure World

The deeper you walk The Purification Principle, the clearer you become, and the more obvious the world's impurities appear. Not just in the air, water, and food, but in the noise, pace, values, and the ways people treat one another.

This clarity is both a gift and a challenge. A gift, because you see truth with unclouded eyes. A challenge, because you cannot unknow what you now know. The question becomes: *How do I remain clear without becoming rigid? How do I hold purity without building a wall between myself and the world?*

To live purity in an impure world is to walk a path of balance, neither retreating into isolation nor surrendering to contamination. You carry an inner flame into the marketplace, the workplace, and the crowded streets, knowing that the light will at times flicker but need not go out. The world will test your clarity with noise, temptations, and constant urgencies, yet these very tests become the training ground where purity matures from fragile ideal into embodied strength.

Purity as an Inner State

Purity is not about living in a bubble and avoiding all contact with the dust of the world. We emphasize being so rooted in your own clarity that you can move through the dust without letting the debris settle in you.

In indigenous traditions, purification ceremonies were not performed once and forgotten. They were repeated often, after travel, after conflict, and after illness, because the people knew that living in the world meant continually brushing off what did not belong.

Your daily and weekly practices are your ongoing ceremonies. They are how you return to your center, no matter what you encounter.

The Art of Selective Immersion

You will not always be in control of your environment. You may travel, attend gatherings, or work in places where food is processed, air is stale, and pace is frantic. The purifier learns the art of selective immersion, engaging fully with what is nourishing in a situation and letting the rest pass through without attachment.

In practice:

• Seek the cleanest water available and carry your own when possible.

• Eat the purest option offered, without turning the meal into a battle of ideals.

• Step outside for air and sunlight whenever you can.

• End the day with a small ritual to reset such as a shower, a glass of lemon water, or a few minutes of breathwork.

Selective immersion is not about withdrawal, but about discernment. We carry the ability to walk through a crowded space without being swept away by currents and to taste what is offered without swallowing what is harmful. Like the lotus rising from mud yet remaining unstained, the purifier learns to engage without absorbing and to move among impurities without letting them take root within. This is a subtle art, requiring both presence and gentleness. A refusal to harden, even as you choose carefully what you allow inside.

Over time, this practice becomes less about what you avoid and more about what you carry with you. The clarity you cultivate acts as a shield, not of rigidity, but of resonance. When your body is well-nourished, mind steady, and spirit grounded, environments of impurity have less power to sway you. You move through them as clean water through stone.

Guarding the Senses

Toxins are not only physical. Impurity enters through what we watch, read, and listen to; through the conversations we linger in; and through the spaces we spend time in.

The purifier chooses input with intention. This does not mean cutting off from reality but choosing reality that strengthens rather than weakens.

• Limit news to what you can act upon, not what will only leave you anxious.

• Curate what you read and watch so the content uplifts, educates, or inspires.

• Keep company with people whose presence feels like clean water.

In the teachings of Thich Nhat Hanh, *"guarding the senses"* is a form of nourishment. Every image, sound, and word is a kind of food for the mind. Choose your diet wisely.

From the moment we are born, our senses are placed under siege. Gloves are placed on our hands to *"protect"* us from the earth's dirt, weakening our skin's dialogue with soil and texture. Glasses are prescribed early and often, not always to correct but to compensate, leaving our natural lens muscles to atrophy rather than strengthen.

The constant roar of traffic and machinery in our cities becomes a form of violence against the ears, drowning out the subtler sounds of wind, birds, or silence. Our tongues are dulled by chemicals hidden in processed food, so that sweetness and salt arrive in toxic excess while nuance and vitality vanish. Even our sense of smell is corrupted by pollution, fragrances, and artificial *"freshness"* that mask rather than reveal.

Yet thought and breath may be the most assaulted, and vital, of all our senses. The breath is meant to be slow and deep, like the tides, yet most of us live in a state of shallow, rapid inhalation, with our nervous systems locked in tension by design. Our thought, once meant to be a tool of wonder and reflection, is now bombarded from every side with advertising, screens, propaganda, and comparison.

To guard the senses is therefore not just to protect what we see, hear, taste, touch, and smell, but to reclaim the sacredness of thought and the rhythm of breath. These are the inner senses that anchor all the others, and when they are tended well, they restore the body's temple to clarity.

Purity in Relationships

You cannot control others' choices, but you can live your values quietly and consistently. The world changes not because we argue our circumstances into submission, but because we embody something better.

When others question your choices, speak from experience, not judgment. Tell your story. Share how you feel, what you have noticed, and how you have healed. Invite curiosity instead of defensiveness.

In indigenous communities, purity was often a collective value. Everyone benefited from clean water, shared meals, and sacred space. You can plant seeds of that same collective purity by offering your home, your table, and your time as examples of what is possible.

Purity in relationships also means practicing discernment with compassion. Some connections will strengthen your flow, while others continually cloud. The purifier learns not to sever with anger but to set boundaries with grace, allowing space where needed while keeping the heart open. In this way, even distance can be an act of love.

Restoring After Exposure

No matter how careful you are, you will encounter toxins. They can be physical, emotional, and energetic. The key is not to fear them, but to have a plan for releasing them quickly.

• Hydrate deeply and add minerals after travel or processed food.

• Use breathwork to calm the nervous system after stressful environments.

• Burn cedar, sage, or incense to clear the energy of your space and self.

• Take an herbal bath or sweat in a sauna to move impurities out through the skin.

Restoration is about detoxing the body while also remembering the body's natural rhythm after having been disrupted. After travel, noise, conflict, or unhealthy food, we can forget that imbalance does not have to linger. The purifier approaches exposure with immediacy and gentleness, tending to the body's rivers before they grow stagnant. Even a few minutes of deep breathing, a glass of Kangen water, or a walk barefoot on the earth can begin the reset. Small acts, performed with intention, send a powerful signal: *you are safe, you are clear, and you can release this now.*

We must also see restoration as ceremony rather than punishment. Too often we react to exposure with guilt, harsh cleansing, or shame, as if impurity were a moral failure. The purifier understands that exposure is inevitable, and recovery is an art. When the reset is honored as sacred, whether through sweat, herbs, frequency therapies, or simply stillness, the body learns to release more quickly each time. In this way, restoration becomes less about repair and more about resilience and strengthening the river to remain clear.

The Quiet Confidence of Purity

Living purity in an impure world is not about withdrawal. This can be explained as being the clear water in the cup, whether you are poured into a mountain spring or traversing a crowded city street.

Over time, you will find that you need less perfection in your surroundings because you have built so much resilience within. You will walk through noise, through crowds, and through the chaos of airports and markets, and still feel the steady current of your own river.

The world will notice. Not because you are loud about your purity, but because clarity has a presence that calms the room and makes people want to know what you know.

In this way, living purity becomes a service. You are no longer just walking The Purification Principle for yourself you are carrying this embodiment into places that may never have known such a thing existed. That, perhaps, is the greatest purification of all.

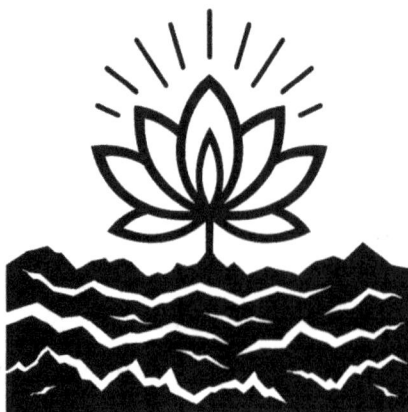

Chapter Twelve: Becoming the River

A river does not think about being pure. She does not set resolutions or track clarity. Her essence is simply to flow. Her nature is removing what does not belong, carrying nourishment where needed, and renewing through constant movement and exchange.

This is the aim of The Purification Principle: *that the practices, the rituals, the choices, and the awareness you have gathered here no longer feel like a program to follow, but like the most natural way to live.*

To become the river is to embody rhythm instead of rigidity. To trust that your body, once unburdened, will choose flow without effort. You will rise and drink because your cells thirst for pure hydration, not because of a checklist. You will breathe deeply because this feels like returning, not because a teacher told you to count your inhales. The practices dissolve into instinct, and instinct is revealed to be the very voice of nature moving through you.

The river does not compare herself to the stream beside her, nor judge her own path when she bends and slows. In the same way, purified life does not chase perfection or pace against another. Seasons of flood and seasons of drought are honored, knowing both are part of the same current. Some days you will feel the water rushing, filled with clarity and strength. Other days the river will move quietly, almost still. Even then, purity remains, hidden beneath the surface, waiting to rise again.

Over time, you will see that your own river is part of a greater watershed. Your clarity nourishes others. Your resilience strengthens the banks of those around you. Your flow becomes an invitation for family, community, and the world to remember that purity is not outside of us, but within.

From Effort to Essence

In the beginning, the work of purification may feel deliberate, even effortful. You choose what to eat and what to avoid. You set aside time for breathwork and movement. You remind yourself to drink water, to rest, to step outside, and to keep your medicine chest stocked.

Over time, though, these essentials become second nature. They stop feeling like practices and start feeling like *you*. The river no longer needs coaxing to run because she remembers her course.

The goal is not to live in constant alignment, not persisted vigilance. You will still encounter interference, perhaps from a fallen branch, or unexpected storm, but instead of clouding for months, you will clear in moments.

The River's Three Truths

As you integrate the Purification Principle into your life, remember the three truths of every healthy river:

• **Know how to release** — A river that clings to her water stagnates. You must continue to let go of what is not yours to carry, whether a toxin, a thought, or a relationship.

• **Know how to receive** — A river is fed by springs, rain, and tributaries. You too must remain open to new sources of nourishment through fresh knowledge, supportive community, and the beauty of the natural world.

• **Know how to adapt** — A river will change course to keep moving toward the sea. You must allow yourself the same flexibility, adjusting your practices and priorities to the seasons of your life.

Living as a Purifier

To live as a purifier is not to retreat from the world's impurities, but to meet them with such clarity that they cannot root in you. You will walk through cities and markets and crowded airports and still feel the steady pulse of your own breath.

You will share meals with family who do not eat as you do and still feel nourished, because your choices are rooted in love, not fear. You will offer your presence as much as your knowledge, understanding that purity is communicated more by how you live than by what you say.

Over time, your life becomes a kind of medicine. An invitation to others to remember their own river. Living this way is to become a still point in a turning world. People will sense something steady in you, a calmness that does not bend to noise, distraction, or chaos. They may not understand your practices, but they will feel the way your presence clears a room without words and offers peace simply by being. Your clarity becomes a silent teaching, a mirror in which others glimpse their own capacity for wholeness.

When challenges rise, whether illness, loss, exhaustion, or conflict, the purifier meets them not as disasters but as currents to be navigated. The practices you have woven into your life will hold you steady, carrying you through hardship without losing your essence. In this, you become a living demonstration that purity is not fragile but resilient, expansive, and strong enough to meet the world as is, while continuing to flow as always meant to.

The Sacred Exchange

In indigenous ways, purification was never just for the individual. The clearer you are, the more you can give to your people, your land, and the future. You are not simply cleaning your own fluids; you are ensuring that the waters that flow from you, being your words, your work, and your creations, are life-giving to others.

When you adapt The Purification Principle, you become part of a larger cycle of restoration. Your vitality nourishes your community. Your clarity influences your choices in business, parenting, and service. Your resilience allows you to meet challenges without passing on more harm.

This exchange is not transactional, but relational. You are not giving to receive; you are giving because your nature is to overflow once your vessel is clear. Just as a spring does not withhold water or measure worth, you learn to pour without fear of depletion. Abundance is scooped from abundance, and yet, abundance remains. In this way, your life becomes prayer in motion. Each act of kindness, all moments of presence, and every instance of offering your gifts is an extension of the river flowing through you.

The Sacred Exchange also means that purification is never only personal but is also ecological. Every time you choose clean food, you support soil that can breathe again. Every time you speak truthfully instead of cynically, you change the atmosphere of a room. Every time you regulate your nervous system before speaking, you prevent ripples of harm from spreading to others. What you cultivate within becomes inseparable from what you create around you.

Perhaps most importantly, this exchange restores belonging. Modern life has trained us to believe we are separated from nature, from community, and from spirit. Yet purification reveals the opposite: *you are a strand in the great web, a current in the great river, and a breath in the great wind.*

Your clarity is not yours alone. This is a gift for those who came before you, for those walking beside you now, and for those yet to come. To live in purity is to live as a bridge, carrying life forward in a way that makes the whole stronger.

The Ongoing Journey

There is no finish line here. Only the ongoing dance of removing, restoring, and rebuilding each day, every season, and in all chapters of your life. Some years you will deepen into advanced practices at places like SoulSpire, layering ozone therapy, Kambo, hyperbaric oxygen, colon hydrotherapy, Rife therapy, and the BioCharger into your renewal. Other years, you will live in the simplicity of garden greens, morning walks, and quiet breathwork. Both are part of the principle. Both diverge into the river.

The journey is not about intensity, but about intimacy and learning to listen more closely to what your body, mind, and spirit are asking for in each season. At times, the call will be for depth and challenge, and at others, for gentleness and ease. The beauty of The Purification Principle is how this adapts with you, meeting you in both your strength and your softness.

Whether through advanced technologies or the simple act of watching the sunrise with steady breath, the river remains the same: *ever-flowing, ever-renewing, ever-carrying you home.*

Your Final Invitation

As you step from these pages back into your daily life, I invite you to see yourself not just as a student of The Purification Principle, but as a living embodiment. Every choice you make, from what you eat and what you think, to how you move and how you speak, is a ripple.

Let those ripples be clear. Let them carry vitality, truth, and beauty downstream. Let them nourish shores you will never see. When your own journey feels heavy or unclear, return to the river. Return to your breath, your water, your plants, and your practices. Remove, restore, and rebuild. Be persistent and consistent, without hurry, and without end.

We learn that purity is not a destination you reach but is the current that carries you home. Know that you do not walk alone. Every purifier who chooses clarity adds strength to the collective current, widening the river for all who come after.

Your quiet devotion becomes part of a greater movement. One that heals families, communities, and the living earth. Step forward not with the weight of obligation, but with the joy of belonging to something vast and eternal: *the river of life, flowing pure and free.*

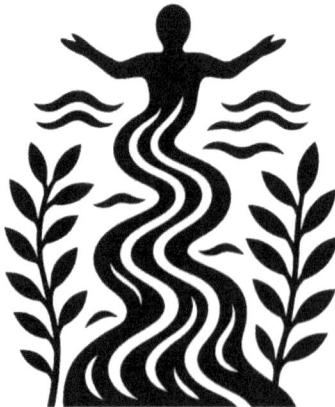

Epilogue: From Our River to Yours

When we began shaping *The Purification Principle*™, we imagined this as more than a book. We wanted the concept to be a companion and complementary resource for the services we offer at Soulspire. Our vision was to represent a voice that walks beside you through the clearings, seasons, and still waters of your own purification.

Every chapter here is drawn from rivers we have each had to wade through ourselves. Some were icy with challenge. Some were warm and easy. All of them taught us the same truth: *purity is not a condition you achieve once and keep forever but is a relationship you tend, like a fire or a garden, day after day.*

As you close these pages, remember:

• You are not expected to be perfect.

• You are not behind.

• You have not missed your chance.

• The river will always welcome you back.

Walk The Purification Principle gently. Let your journey be less about rigid rules and more about remembering who you are without the interference, the stagnation, and the noise. Rekindle a friendship with your body, with the plants, with the seasons, and with the unseen currents that have been guiding you all along.

We are honored to have shared this journey with you, not as authorities standing on the shore, but as fellow travelers in the water. May your flow be steady, your banks be strong, and the clarity you cultivate ripple outward, nourishing shores you will never see.

About the Authors

Jesse Jacoby is a dedicated father and founder and CEO of Soulspire: The Healing Playground (*soulspire.com*). This is a biohacking and purification center with locations near Lake Tahoe in Truckee, CA, and in Nevada City, CA. The Soulspire Retreat home is located in West Hollywood, CA.

Additionally, Jesse is a co-founder of Substance Shield (substanceshield.com), which is an organic, wild-crafted supplement line for replenishing the body before and after substance use.

Jesse is the author of The Raw Cure: Healing Beyond Medicine (1st & 2nd Editions), The Way Knows: Trusting Divine Orchestration, Where Galaxies Kiss the Earth, The High Life, Windsdom: Wisdom from the Wind, Sovereign Biology, Immune to Fatigue, Modern Human Conditions, You Are Not Powerless, Forged: The Twelve Foundations of Manhood, Gaia Speaks, Eating Plant-Based: The New Health Paradigm, & My Quest to Conquer What Matters.

He also co-founded Little Manifestors Publishing and has authored over thirty children's books.

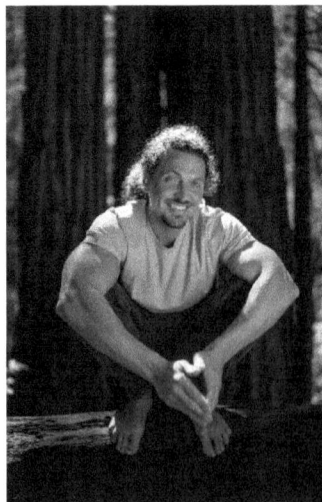

Sydney Thackray is a multi-genre author, filmmaker, and entrepreneur whose work explores the intersection of spirit, strategy, and storytelling. Whether crafting lyrical children's tales that uplift the soul or publishing visionary guides for wellness and business, Sydney writes to awaken potential in readers of all ages.

A Dame of the Saint Martin Order, she has studied spiritual traditions across the globe, from the Druids of Stonehenge to the energy healers of Bali and has spoken at wellness and consciousness events including the LA Conscious Life Expo. Her experience spans clean technology, humanitarian work, and media, including her upcoming feature film, supplement company, Substance Shield™, and biohacking center, Soulspire: The Healing Playground.

No matter the form, Sydney's writing is grounded in purpose: to inspire clarity, compassion, and courageous action in a complex world.

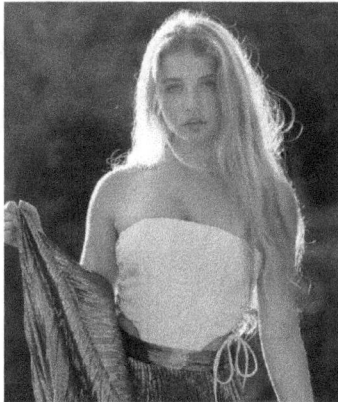

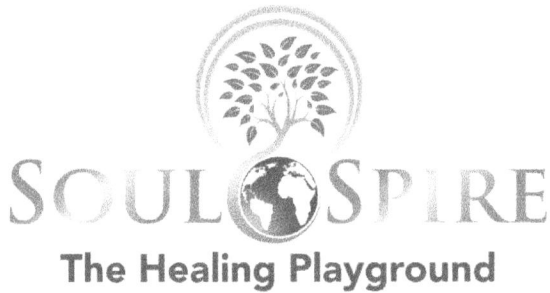

SOUL🌍SPIRE
The Healing Playground

Soulspire is a biohacking and purification offering with centers located in Truckee, CA, and Nevada City, CA which provides each of the biohacking tools suggested in this guide for regenerating the body before and after substance use.

Access the site www.soulspire.com

Substance Shield
Ally of the Aftermath

Substance Shield is a botanical supplement line born from the wisdom of The High Life, a guide for conscious living in a chemically saturated world. Our products exist to support the body's resilience before and after exposure to substances, offering tools of renewal, not judgment. Whether facing pharmaceutical fallout, recreational recovery, or environmental residue, our mission is to replenish what modern life strips away.

Every formula is organic, vegan, wild-harvested, and crafted from whole foods, roots, and ancient botanicals designed to support detoxification pathways, restore depleted micronutrients, and aid in cellular resilience.

Our Mission

• To honor the human experience without shame.

• To offer nourishment to those navigating a chemically compromised world.

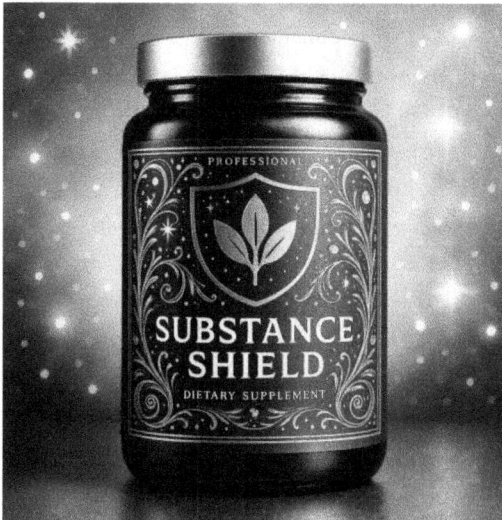

www.substanceshield.com

Bibliography

Introduction:

Bailey, Alice A. *Initiation, Human and Solar*. Lucis Publishing, 1922.

Chopra, Deepak. *Ageless Body, Timeless Mind: The Quantum Alternative to Growing Old*. Harmony Books, 1993.

Hanh, Thich Nhat. *Peace Is Every Step: The Path of Mindfulness in Everyday Life*. Bantam, 1991.

Rudd, Richard. *The Gene Keys: Embracing Your Higher Purpose*. Eden, 2013.

Trungpa, Chögyam. *Cutting Through Spiritual Materialism*. Shambhala Publications, 1973.

Chapter I:

Berceli, David. *The Revolutionary Trauma Release Process: Transcend Your Toughest Times*. Namaste Publishing, 2008.

Campbell, Joseph. *The Hero with a Thousand Faces*. Princeton University Press, 1949.

Challem, Jack. *Feed Your Genes Right: Eat to Turn Off Disease-Causing Bad Genes and Turn On the Good Ones for Health and Longevity*. Wiley, 2006.

Hanh, Thich Nhat. *The Miracle of Mindfulness: An Introduction to the Practice of Meditation*. Beacon Press, 1975.

Katz, Sandor Ellix. *Wild Fermentation: The Flavor, Nutrition, and Craft of Live-Culture Foods*. Chelsea Green Publishing, 2017.

Miller, Iva, and Arkan Lushwala. *Time of the Black Jaguar: An Offering of Indigenous Wisdom for the Continuity of Life on Earth*. Findhorn Press, 2011.

Myers, Natasha. *Rendering Life Molecular: Models, Modelers, and Excitable Matter*. Duke University Press, 2015.

Noble, Vicki. *Shakti Woman: Feeling Our Fire, Healing Our World*. HarperOne, 1991.

Rossi, Ernest L., and David Lloyd. *The Psychobiology of Gene Expression: Neuroscience and Neurogenesis in Hypnosis and the Healing Arts*. W. W. Norton & Company, 1992.

Siegel, Daniel J. *The Developing Mind: How Relationships and the Brain Interact to Shape Who We Are*. Guilford Press, 1999.

Wallace, B. Alan. *The Attention Revolution: Unlocking the Power of the Focused Mind*. Wisdom Publications, 2006.

Chapter II:

Atwood, Kim. *Sacred Smoke: The Ancient Art of Smudging for Modern Times*. Sterling Ethos, 2019.

Bailey, Eric, and Robin W. Kimmerer. *Braiding Sweetgrass: Indigenous Wisdom, Scientific Knowledge, and the Teachings of Plants*. Milkweed Editions, 2013.

Buhner, Stephen Harrod. *Sacred Plant Medicine: Explorations in the Practice of Indigenous Herbalism*. Bear & Company, 1996.

Caldecott, Todd. *Ayurveda: The Divine Science of Life*. Elsevier, 2006.

Colbin, Annemarie. *Food and Healing: How What You Eat Determines Your Health, Your Well-Being, and the Quality of Your Life*. Ballantine Books, 1986.

Gittleman, Ann Louise. *Living Beauty Detox Program: The Revolutionary Diet for Each and Every Season of a Woman's Life*. HarperOne, 2000.

Harner, Michael. *The Way of the Shaman*. Harper & Row, 1980.

Kearney, Michael. *Mortally Wounded: Stories of Soul Pain, Death, and Healing*. Scribner, 1996.

Kearney, Margaret. *Healing Circles: Grief Rituals and the Restoration of Connection*. Inner Traditions, 2005.

Pitchford, Paul. *Healing with Whole Foods: Asian Traditions and Modern Nutrition*. North Atlantic Books, 2002.

Roszak, Theodore. *The Voice of the Earth: An Exploration of Ecopsychology*. Simon & Schuster, 1992.

Weil, Andrew. *Spontaneous Healing: How to Discover and Embrace Your Body's Natural Ability to Maintain and Heal Itself*. Knopf, 1995.

Chapter III:

Batmanghelidj, Fereydoon. *Your Body's Many Cries for Water: You Are Not Sick, You Are Thirsty! Don't Treat Thirst with Medications*. Global Health Solutions, 1997.

Brown, Bessel van der Kolk. *The Body Keeps the Score: Brain, Mind, and Body in the Healing of Trauma*. Viking, 2014.

Campbell, Stuart. *Energy Medicine: The Science and Mystery of Healing*. North Atlantic Books, 2019.

Chia, Mantak. *Awaken Healing Energy Through the Tao: The Taoist Secret of Circulating Internal Power*. Aurora Press, 1983.

Cousins, Norman. *Anatomy of an Illness as Perceived by the Patient*. Norton, 1979.

Herbert, Benson. *The Relaxation Response*. HarperTorch, 1975.

Naviaux, Robert K. "Metabolic Features of the Cell Danger Response." *Mitochondrion*, vol. 16, 2014, pp. 7–17.

Pollack, Gerald H. *The Fourth Phase of Water: Beyond Solid, Liquid, and Vapor*. Ebner and Sons, 2013.

Satchidananda, Swami. *The Yoga Sutras of Patanjali*. Integral Yoga Publications, 1978.

Stone, Michael. *Yoga for a World Out of Balance: Teachings on Ethics and Social Action*. Shambhala, 2009.

Thurman, Robert A. F. *Inner Revolution: Life, Liberty, and the Pursuit of Real Happiness*. Riverhead Books, 1998.

Wallace, B. Alan. *The Attention Revolution: Unlocking the Power of the Focused Mind*. Wisdom Publications, 2006.

Chapter IV:

Attwood, Angela. *Adaptogens: Herbs for Strength, Stamina, and Stress Relief*. Healing Arts Press, 2019.

Bennett, Brian J., and Rob Knight. *The Microbiome and Human Health: Beyond the Gut*. Nature Reviews Genetics, vol. 21, 2020, pp. 581–96.

Buhner, Stephen Harrod. *Herbal Antibiotics: Natural Alternatives for Treating Drug-Resistant Bacteria*. Storey Publishing, 2012.

Campbell, Bruce, and Michael F. Holick. *Vitamin D: Physiology, Molecular Biology, and Clinical Applications*. Humana Press, 2019.

Carroll, Sean, et al. *Mitochondria and the Future of Medicine: The Key to Understanding Disease, Chronic Illness, Aging, and Life Itself*. Chelsea Green Publishing, 2018.

Challem, Jack. *The Inflammation Syndrome: Your Nutrition Plan for Great Health, Weight Loss, and Pain-Free Living*. Wiley, 2003.

Guggenheimer, Eva. *The Rainbow Diet: Plant Colors as Medicine*. Findhorn Press, 2002.

Harner, Michael. *The Way of the Shaman*. Harper & Row, 1980.

Kimmerer, Robin Wall. *Braiding Sweetgrass: Indigenous Wisdom, Scientific Knowledge, and the Teachings of Plants*. Milkweed Editions, 2013.

Natelson, Benjamin H. *Stress Response Syndromes: PTSD, Grief, and Adjustment Disorders*. Guilford Press, 2010.

Naviaux, Robert K. "Metabolic Features of the Cell Danger Response." *Mitochondrion*, vol. 16, 2014, pp. 7–17.

Pitchford, Paul. *Healing with Whole Foods: Asian Traditions and Modern Nutrition*. North Atlantic Books, 2002.

Rothschild, Babette. *The Body Remembers: The Psychophysiology of Trauma and Trauma Treatment*. Norton, 2000.

Sapolsky, Robert M. *Why Zebras Don't Get Ulcers: The Acclaimed Guide to Stress, Stress-Related Diseases, and Coping*. Holt Paperbacks, 2004.

Seifert, John G., et al. "Cold Water Immersion and Exercise Recovery: Effects on Health and Performance." *Journal of Physiology*, vol. 594, no. 18, 2016, pp. 5205–16.

Wallace, David R. *The Healing Power of Adaptogens: The Best Herbs for Fighting Stress and Restoring Health*. Storey Publishing, 2020.

Chapter V:

Andrews, Ted. *Animal-Speak: The Spiritual & Magical Powers of Creatures Great & Small*. Llewellyn Publications, 1993.

Bopp, Judie, et al. *The Sacred Tree*. Four Worlds International Institute, 1989.

Buhner, Stephen Harrod. *Plant Intelligence and the Imaginal Realm: Beyond the Doors of Perception into the Dreaming of Earth*. Bear & Company, 2014.

Chopra, Deepak. *The Seven Spiritual Laws of Success: A Practical Guide to the Fulfillment of Your Dreams*. New World Library, 1994.

Halifax, Joan. *The Fruitful Darkness: A Journey Through Buddhist Practice and Tribal Wisdom*. Grove Press, 1993.

Hanh, Thich Nhat. *Silence: The Power of Quiet in a World Full of Noise*. HarperOne, 2015.

Kimmerer, Robin Wall. *Braiding Sweetgrass: Indigenous Wisdom, Scientific Knowledge, and the Teachings of Plants*. Milkweed Editions, 2013.

Meadows, Donella H. *Thinking in Systems: A Primer*. Chelsea Green Publishing, 2008.

Rinpoche, Sogyal. *The Tibetan Book of Living and Dying*. HarperSanFrancisco, 1992.

Stone, Michael. *Yoga for a World Out of Balance: Teachings on Ethics and Social Action*. Shambhala Publications, 2009.

Tacey, David. *ReEnchantment: The New Australian Spirituality*. HarperCollins, 2000.

Chapter VI:

Anderson, E. N. *Everyone Eats: Understanding Food and Culture*. NYU Press, 2005.

Buhner, Stephen Harrod. *Sacred Plant Medicine: Explorations in the Practice of Indigenous Herbalism*. Bear & Company, 1996.

Colbin, Annemarie. *Food and Healing: How What You Eat Determines Your Health, Your Well-Being, and the Quality of Your Life*. Ballantine Books, 1986.

Guggenheimer, Eva. *The Rainbow Diet: Plant Colors as Medicine*. Findhorn Press, 2002.

Katz, Sandor Ellix. *Wild Fermentation: The Flavor, Nutrition, and Craft of Live-Culture Foods*. Chelsea Green Publishing, 2017.

Kimmerer, Robin Wall. *Braiding Sweetgrass: Indigenous Wisdom, Scientific Knowledge, and the Teachings of Plants*. Milkweed Editions, 2013.

Pitchford, Paul. *Healing with Whole Foods: Asian Traditions and Modern Nutrition*. North Atlantic Books, 2002.

Pollan, Michael. *In Defense of Food: An Eater's Manifesto*. Penguin, 2008.

Rozin, Paul. "The Meaning of Food in Our Lives: A Cross-Cultural Perspective on Eating and Well-Being." *Journal of Nutrition Education and Behavior*, vol. 39, no. 2, 2007, pp. 121–25.

Schlosser, Eric. *Fast Food Nation: The Dark Side of the All-American Meal*. Houghton Mifflin, 2001.

Shiva, Vandana. *Staying Alive: Women, Ecology, and Development*. Zed Books, 2010.

Chapter VII:

Buhner, Stephen Harrod. *Herbal Antibiotics: Natural Alternatives for Treating Drug-Resistant Bacteria*. Storey Publishing, 2012.

Buhner, Stephen Harrod. *Sacred Plant Medicine: Explorations in the Practice of Indigenous Herbalism*. Bear & Company, 1996.

Chevallier, Andrew. *Encyclopedia of Herbal Medicine*. DK Publishing, 2016.

Gladstar, Rosemary. *Rosemary Gladstar's Herbal Recipes for Vibrant Health: 175 Teas, Tonics, Oils, Salves, Tinctures, and Other Natural Remedies for the Entire Family*. Storey Publishing, 2001.

Hoffmann, David. *Medical Herbalism: The Science and Practice of Herbal Medicine*. Healing Arts Press, 2003.

Kimmerer, Robin Wall. *Braiding Sweetgrass: Indigenous Wisdom, Scientific Knowledge, and the Teachings of Plants*. Milkweed Editions, 2013.

Mars, Brigitte. *The Desktop Guide to Herbal Medicine: The Ultimate Multidisciplinary Reference to Nature's Botanicals*. McGraw-Hill, 2007.

McIntyre, Anne. *The Complete Woman's Herbal: A Manual of Healing Herbs and Nutrition for Personal Well-Being and Family Care*. Henry Holt, 1994.

Moore, Michael. *Medicinal Plants of the Pacific West*. Museum of New Mexico Press, 1993.

Pitchford, Paul. *Healing with Whole Foods: Asian Traditions and Modern Nutrition*. North Atlantic Books, 2002.

Ross, Gordon. *Reishi Mushroom: Herb of Spiritual Potency and Medical Wonder*. Kensington, 1999.

Shiva, Vandana. *Staying Alive: Women, Ecology, and Development*. Zed Books, 2010.

Tierra, Michael. *The Way of Herbs*. Pocket Books, 1998.

Valerie, Ann Worwood. *The Complete Book of Essential Oils and Aromatherapy*. New World Library, 1991.

Chapter VIII:

Benson, Herbert. *The Relaxation Response*. HarperTorch, 1975.

Buhner, Stephen Harrod. *Plant Intelligence and the Imaginal Realm: Beyond the Doors of Perception into the Dreaming of Earth*. Bear & Company, 2014.

Campbell, Stuart. *Energy Medicine: The Science and Mystery of Healing*. North Atlantic Books, 2019.

Chia, Mantak. *Awaken Healing Energy Through the Tao: The Taoist Secret of Circulating Internal Power*. Aurora Press, 1983.

Farb, Peter, and George Armelagos. *Consuming Passions: The Anthropology of Eating*. Houghton Mifflin, 1980.

Gladstar, Rosemary. *Herbal Healing for Women: Simple Home Remedies for Women of All Ages*. Touchstone, 1993.

Gregg, Braden. *Walking Between the Worlds: The Science of Compassion*. Radio Bookstore Press, 1997.

Hanh, Thich Nhat. *Silence: The Power of Quiet in a World Full of Noise*. HarperOne, 2015.

Hanh, Thich Nhat. *Peace Is Every Step: The Path of Mindfulness in Everyday Life*. Bantam, 1991.

Kearney, Michael. *Mortally Wounded: Stories of Soul Pain, Death, and Healing*. Scribner, 1996.

Kimmerer, Robin Wall. *Braiding Sweetgrass: Indigenous Wisdom, Scientific Knowledge, and the Teachings of Plants*. Milkweed Editions, 2013.

Naviaux, Robert K. "Metabolic Features of the Cell Danger Response." *Mitochondrion*, vol. 16, 2014, pp. 7–17.

Pitchford, Paul. *Healing with Whole Foods: Asian Traditions and Modern Nutrition*. North Atlantic Books, 2002.

Rothschild, Babette. *The Body Remembers: The Psychophysiology of Trauma and Trauma Treatment*. Norton, 2000.

Stone, Michael. *Yoga for a World Out of Balance: Teachings on Ethics and Social Action*. Shambhala, 2009.

Chapter IX:

Bopp, Judie, et al. *The Sacred Tree*. Four Worlds International Institute, 1989.

Caldecott, Todd. *Ayurveda: The Divine Science of Life*. Elsevier, 2006.

Cowan, Thomas. *The Fourfold Path to Healing: Working with the Laws of Nutrition, Therapeutics, Movement and Meditation in the Art of Medicine*. New Trends Publishing, 2004.

Frawley, David. *Ayurveda and the Mind: The Healing of Consciousness*. Lotus Press, 1997.

Gladstar, Rosemary. *Herbal Healing for Men and Women: Simple Home Remedies Using Herbs, Teas, and Natural Foods*. Fireside, 1993.

Halifax, Joan. *The Fruitful Darkness: A Journey Through Buddhist Practice and Tribal Wisdom*. Grove Press, 1993.

Hoppál, Mihály. *Shamanism: An Introduction*. International Society for Shamanistic Research, 2007.

Katz, Sandor Ellix. *The Art of Fermentation: An In-Depth Exploration of Essential Concepts and Processes from Around the World*. Chelsea Green Publishing, 2012.

Kimmerer, Robin Wall. *Braiding Sweetgrass: Indigenous Wisdom, Scientific Knowledge, and the Teachings of Plants*. Milkweed Editions, 2013.

Pitchford, Paul. *Healing with Whole Foods: Asian Traditions and Modern Nutrition*. North Atlantic Books, 2002.

Ross, Gordon. *Reishi Mushroom: Herb of Spiritual Potency and Medical Wonder*. Kensington, 1999.

Wallace, B. Alan. *The Attention Revolution: Unlocking the Power of the Focused Mind*. Wisdom Publications, 2006.

Chapter X:

Achterberg, Jeanne. *Imagery in Healing: Shamanism and Modern Medicine*. Shambhala Publications, 1985.

Atkinson, Roland F. *Colon Hydrotherapy: Principles, Equipment, and Applications*. CRC Press, 2013.

Buhner, Stephen Harrod. *Sacred Plant Medicine: Explorations in the Practice of Indigenous Herbalism*. Bear & Company, 1996.

Caldecott, Todd. *Ayurveda: The Divine Science of Life*. Elsevier, 2006.

Chia, Mantak. *Chi Nei Tsang: Internal Organs Chi Massage*. Destiny Books, 2007.

Csordas, Thomas J. *The Sacred Self: A Cultural Phenomenology of Charismatic Healing*. University of California Press, 1997.

Glatthaar-Saalmüller, Brigitte. "Ozone Therapy and Its Scientific Foundations." *Journal of Natural Science, Biology and Medicine*, vol. 9, no. 1, 2018, pp. 20–28.

Goodman, Felicitas D. *Where the Spirits Ride the Wind: Trance Journeys and Other Ecstatic Experiences*. Indiana University Press, 1990.

Halifax, Joan. *The Fruitful Darkness: A Journey Through Buddhist Practice and Tribal Wisdom*. Grove Press, 1993.

Kambo, Peter Gorman. *Sapo in My Soul: The Matsés Frog Medicine*. Icaro Publishing, 2015.

Kellogg, John Harvey. *Colon Hygiene: Nature's Way to Health*. Modern Medicine Publishing, 1917.

Moss, David. *Hyperbaric Oxygen Therapy: A Clinical Guide*. Best Publishing, 2019.

Pollack, Gerald H. *The Fourth Phase of Water: Beyond Solid, Liquid, and Vapor*. Ebner and Sons, 2013.

Rife, Royal Raymond. *The Cancer Cure That Worked: Fifty Years of Suppression*. New Century Press, 1987.

Sadhguru. *Body: The Greatest Gadget*. Isha Foundation, 2010.

Stevenson, Ninian. *The Sweat Lodge: Native American Ceremonial Healing*. Inner Traditions, 2006.

Tachibana, Hiroshi. "Effects of Hyperbaric Oxygen Therapy on Inflammation and Healing." *Medical Gas Research*, vol. 6, no. 4, 2016, pp. 216–23.

Wahbeh, Helané, et al. "Sound Healing and the Use of Singing Bowls: A Systematic Review." *Journal of Evidence-Based Integrative Medicine*, vol. 22, no. 4, 2017, pp. 788–96.

Weil, Andrew. *Spontaneous Healing: How to Discover and Embrace Your Body's Natural Ability to Maintain and Heal Itself*. Knopf, 1995.

Chapter XI:

Abram, David. *The Spell of the Sensuous: Perception and Language in a More-Than-Human World*. Vintage, 1996.

Bai, Tian Dayton. *Emotional Sobriety: From Relationship Trauma to Resilience and Balance*. Health Communications, 2008.

Bopp, Judie, et al. *The Sacred Tree*. Four Worlds International Institute, 1989.

Hanh, Thich Nhat. *Peace Is Every Step: The Path of Mindfulness in Everyday Life*. Bantam, 1991.

Hanh, Thich Nhat. *Silence: The Power of Quiet in a World Full of Noise*. HarperOne, 2015.

Illich, Ivan. *Medical Nemesis: The Expropriation of Health*. Pantheon, 1976.

Kimmerer, Robin Wall. *Braiding Sweetgrass: Indigenous Wisdom, Scientific Knowledge, and the Teachings of Plants*. Milkweed Editions, 2013.

Maté, Gabor. *When the Body Says No: Exploring the Stress-Disease Connection*. Vintage Canada, 2003.

Miller, Rupert G., et al. *Air Pollution and Public Health: Emerging Hazards and Improved Understanding*. Springer, 2015.

Roszak, Theodore. *The Voice of the Earth: An Exploration of Ecopsychology*. Simon & Schuster, 1992.

Sacks, Oliver. *Musicophilia: Tales of Music and the Brain*. Knopf, 2007.

Smith, Huston. *The World's Religions*. HarperOne, 1991.

Chapter XII:

Abram, David. *The Spell of the Sensuous: Perception and Language in a More-Than-Human World*. Vintage, 1996.

Berry, Thomas. *The Great Work: Our Way into the Future*. Bell Tower, 1999.

Bopp, Judie, et al. *The Sacred Tree*. Four Worlds International Institute, 1989.

Chopra, Deepak. *Ageless Body, Timeless Mind: The Quantum Alternative to Growing Old*. Harmony Books, 1993.

Hanh, Thich Nhat. *The Heart of Understanding: Commentaries on the Prajnaparamita Heart Sutra*. Parallax Press, 1988.

Halifax, Joan. *Standing at the Edge: Finding Freedom Where Fear and Courage Meet*. Flatiron Books, 2018.

Kimmerer, Robin Wall. *Braiding Sweetgrass: Indigenous Wisdom, Scientific Knowledge, and the Teachings of Plants*. Milkweed Editions, 2013.

Lushwala, Arkan. *Time of the Black Jaguar: An Offering of Indigenous Wisdom for the Continuity of Life on Earth*. Findhorn Press, 2011.

Maté, Gabor. *The Myth of Normal: Trauma, Illness, and Healing in a Toxic Culture*. Avery, 2022.

Rudd, Richard. *The Gene Keys: Embracing Your Higher Purpose*. Eden, 2013.

Trungpa, Chögyam. *Sacred Path of the Warrior*. Shambhala Publications, 1984.